The Fundamentals of Science for Nurses

The Fundamentals of Science for Nurses

Cynthia J. Harris BA, RGN, RM, OHNC

with a Foreword by
P. D. Holgate

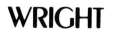

London Boston
Durban Singapore Sydney Toronto Wellington

John Wright

is an imprint of Butterworth Scientific

First published 1988

© **Butterworth & Co. (Publishers) Ltd, 1988**
Borough Green, Sevenoaks, Kent TN15 8PH England

*British Library Cataloguing
in Publication Data*

Harris, Cynthia J.
   The fundamentals of science for nurses.
   1. Nurses   2. Science
   I. Title
   502'.4613   RT69
   ISBN 0-7236-0856-3

Typeset by KEYTEC, Bridport, Dorset

Printed in Great Britain by
Billing and Sons Ltd, Worcester

Preface

It is often not until nurses undertake a post-registration course that involves the study at an advanced level of topics such as physiology, toxicology, clinical conditions and their causes, that a lack of understanding of science subjects becomes a hindrance. Those nurses who have studied physics, chemistry or biology to 'O' level, and the few who have studied these topics to 'A' level, may not experience any difficulties. However, a large percentage of nurses will have done neither and this book aims to help them remedy this problem.

I would emphasize at the outset that this is not intended to be a textbook of physiology, toxicology, biology or any other specific topic related to nursing in its widest context. It can perhaps best be described as a reference work covering some aspects of physics and chemistry which will enable the student to undertake with confidence the study of topics specifically related to any particular nursing specialty.

It is intended that this book should provide a basic foundation on which a deeper and broader knowledge can be built. The topics included are interdependent; indeed it is often difficult to understand one without some knowledge of another. For instance, to understand electricity (Chapter 6) some knowledge of atomic structure (Chapter 4) is necessary, so it would seem logical for atomic structure to appear first. However, to understand the structure of the atom, some knowledge of electricity is needed. Bearing this in mind, topics have been presented in what I consider to be a logical sequence but I accept that what is logical to one person may not be so to another. Where necessary I have referred the reader to a preceding or subsequent chapter. Words whose scientific meaning may not be clear are listed in the Glossary. Explanations of measurements, chemical symbols and some mathematical information will be found in a series of appendices and thus do not clutter the text.

In nursing today there are very many specialties. For this reason examples relating the text to nursing have been kept general rather than specific to any specialty, as have references to the normal living human. As this book has been written with the occupational health nurse in mind, however, there will, perhaps inevitably, be a hint of bias towards this speciality. If this is so, I offer no apology.

Any science subject, particularly to those with no scientific bent, does not lend itself easily to light 'bedside' reading. As far as possible I have tried to present the text in an accessible form. I hope this book will encourage in the reader an awareness of the microscopic world and thus lead to a deeper understanding of the world more readily visible with the naked eye.

C.J.H.

Contents

Foreword

By **P. D. Holgate**

Member, English National Board for Nursing,
Midwifery and Health Visiting,
and
Principal Advisory Tutor in Occupational Health Nursing,
Royal College of Nursing

In today's technological world all nurses need some understanding of science in order to be effective practitioners working from a good knowledge base. Occupational health nurses require a knowledge of the clinical effects of disease and a scientific understanding of the work environment. This book is thus targeted at, but not exclusively orientated to, occupational health nurses. Other groups of nurses are finding that knowledge of the social sciences only is not sufficient to practise, and therefore this book will be a useful tool in every nursing library.

As a former occupational health nurse tutor Cynthia Harris has an understanding of the knowledge deficit in science matters among students following the Occupational Health Nursing Certificate, an understanding equally shared by tutors at all the approved colleges providing the programme.

Science has so many facets, and this book attempts to cover as many as possible without giving the reader mental indigestion, Cynthia Harris, writing with her easy style, is to be congratulated on tackling the topic and making a welcome contribution to the knowledge base of all nurses.

1

Introduction

We tend to view familiar objects in the world around us, both animate and inanimate objects, without consciously thinking what they are made of or what makes them appear in a particular shape or form. True, nurses will tend to think beyond what can be seen with the naked eye as far as a human being is concerned, thinking in terms of a collection of systems each composed of one or more organs, for example the digestive system, composed of mouth, oesophagus, stomach, large and small intestines. Furthermore they will see each organ as a compilation of two or more types of tissue, such as muscle or connective tissue, which in turn is made up of innumerable microscopic structures called cells.

But beyond that each cell is itself a very complex structure, comprised of the protoplasm (living contents) surrounded by a membrane. There are two distinct forms of protoplasm, the nucleus, which contains the genetic material deoxyribonucleic acid (DNA), and the cytoplasm, which contains the material necessary for cell metabolism (*see* Chapter 2). The plasma membrane surrounding the protoplasm controls the flow of material into and out of the cell as well as separating it from other cells.

The cell is the smallest discrete unit of any living organism, animal or plant, and each cell is in itself a complex manufacturing unit. It can be broken down further into its constituent chemicals, because all organisms, including human beings, are no more than a collection of a few solid chemicals and rather a lot of water. And chemicals, in fact everything that exists in the universe, are made up of elements.

There exist a finite number of elements and everything, living and non-living, is made up of elements either in their pure form or in combination with other elements. An atom (*see* Chapter 4) is the smallest particle of an element which can participate in a chemical reaction. However, atoms do not combine in a random manner, they do so only in accordance with certain laws of chemistry and physics. There is nothing special about the atoms which make up living things; for example, the carbon atoms found in all living things are structurally exactly the same as those found in a lump of coal or in a diamond. Nor is there anything magical about the chemistry of living organisms, although the chemical structures found in the human body, that is the biological molecules, are by far the most complex structures in existence in the known universe. Even so, these molecules and the atoms of which they are composed are all governed by the same laws of physics and chemistry as any other substance.

Organisms and their Environment

Some life forms are unicellular, for example bacteria, some viruses and some moulds. Unicellular organisms perform all of the activities necessary for life and reproduction within this one cell. By contrast, an adult male human may be composed of as many as $100\,000\,000\,000$ (10^{11}) cells. All of these will be made up of the same basic chemicals but the cells of different organs and tissues will differ slightly in both structure and function. The major advantage that multicellular organisms have is that they are less dependent on their environment than are unicellular organisms.

Living organisms survive only within a specific and narrow range of physical and chemical conditions. For example, the human body must be maintained at a temperature of about 37 °C (98 °F) and the pH of the blood at approximately 7·4. Any deviations above or below normal limits can have adverse effects and may not be compatible with life. Living organisms have built-in systems by which certain physical and chemical conditions can be regulated. For instance, heat is produced in the human body by the *chemical process* of oxidation and can be lost by the *physical processes* of radiation, convection, condensation and conduction (*see* Chapter 7).

The Rise of Science
Man has evolved as the most intelligent of animals and by the application of scientific method, that is through observation, measurement and experiment, he has discovered some of the laws that govern the workings of the universe. Man therefore has an advantage over other animals; he has the ability both to control and exploit his environment. Greater advances in the realms of science and technology have been made this century than in any other period of history. Twentieth century man is increasingly dependent on man-made systems for power, manufacture, transport, communication etc. Generally this fact is taken very much for granted and the extent and speed of innovations is not consciously appreciated. It does no harm to pause occasionally and to remind ourselves of man's achievements.

Consider, for instance, that the distance travelled by the first powered aeroplane (the Wright brothers' biplane in 1903) was 120 feet, just over half the length of a modern Boeing 747 jumbo jet which has a travelling range of 3500 miles and a carrying capacity of almost 500 passengers. Similarly, the technology which the contemporary nurse takes for granted would surely overwhelm the nurse of 1903. Technology will continue to advance and further scientific discoveries will be made. Today's nurse has a need, if not a duty, to acquire some understanding of the fundamentals of the sciences in order to keep abreast of these discoveries and inventions.

Man's understanding of the world has increased immeasurably since the days of antiquity when responsibility for all events was assigned to gods, who received both credit and blame. When man first began to question the credibility of gods who indiscriminately hurled thunderbolts about the skies, and the intelligence of those who believed in them, the infant science was born. Only when the absolute power of the gods was questioned could man hope to begin to understand either himself or his world.

Modern science is said to have been born in the sixteenth century and since the Industrial Revolution, which began in Britain in the late seventeenth century, the depth of scientific knowledge has increased enormously. (The number of scientists has doubled every ten years since 1700.) Until the eighteenth century, what is now a whole series of specialties was treated as a single subject and called 'natural philosophy'. A trend towards specialization began near the end of that century when a differentiation between chemistry and physics first became recognizable. Today the sciences can be broadly divided into two categories, the physical sciences and the biological sciences.

The physical sciences, which are concerned with the properties and behaviour of non-living matter, can further be divided into two main sections—physics and chemistry. Physics is the science concerned with the properties of matter and the laws of physics are applicable to the world and everything in it, including human beings. These laws are also applicable to the whole universe and to outer space, which is currently being explored and exploited by man. The practical applications of physics have allowed the development of the technology without which today's world could not exist.

Chemistry is the science concerned with the composition of matter, the atoms of which elements are composed and the ways in which they react and combine.

Biochemistry is the science concerned with living things and with the chemical composition of living matter. It is the branch of science that has expanded, and continues to expand, more rapidly than any other. Modern technology and modern techniques are making possible discoveries of immense importance.

Take for instance the discovery of the structure of DNA in 1953 by Crich and Watson (*see* Watson, 1968), which has proved to be one of the greatest scientific events of this century.

Nurses and Science

Today many specialties and sub-specialties exist and those branches of science which are of particular interest to nurses fall into three broad categories—physics, chemistry and biochemistry. The human body is a complex chemical structure whose functions are equally complex. Interaction with the environment serves only to increase this complexity. The intricate interrelationships of composition and activity make study difficult and some knowledge of these basic sciences is essential if nurses are to understand the structure and function of the body and how it reacts and interacts with the diverse environmental conditions in which people live, work and play. For the occupational health nurse this knowledge will facilitate a deeper understanding of the different environmental conditions to be found in places of work. This should help in the identification and control of potentially dangerous situations.

Physiology is of particular interest because the internal function of the human body can be affected by chemicals—including medicines and toxic substances—and by physical conditions such as temperature, radiation and noise.

By thinking beyond the macroscopic world, the world that can be seen with the naked eye, to the activities that occur at the microscopic level, the effects of various conditions and substances on the human body will be more readily understood. The maxim on which this book is based is 'Think microscopic'.

Reference

Watson, J. D. *The Double Helix*. London, Weidenfeld & Nicolson, 1968; Harmondsworth, Penguin, 1970.

2

Energy and motion

In the scientific world many everyday words are assigned specific meanings. 'Work' is such a word. It might be defined in many ways depending upon an individual's conception of what work is. For example, to some it may mean paid employment, to others physical as opposed to mental activity. Still others would consider that leisure activities and sports are definitely not work, yet they are the means whereby many people earn a living.

To define work simply, as do physicists, as the transfer of energy from one physical system to another gives the word a much more precise definition. It can be defined mathematically as:

work = force × distance moved in the direction
of the force

It also provides a definition which indicates the close relationship between work and energy. The word 'energy' is in fact derived from the Greek word *energia* meaning 'active' or 'at work'. Anything which can do work is said to possess energy. Energy can therefore be defined as the capacity to do work.

The unit of measurement for both work and energy is the joule (J).

Energy

When we talk of work we tend to think of some sort of physical exertion or of tasks performed by machine and equipment with greater potential physical and mental power than that possessed by human beings or animals. But the activity of a single atom, that is the attraction between particles within the nucleus of the atom and the attraction between the nucleus and its cloud of electrons (*see* Chapter 4) also involves work, as do the chemical reactions (*see* Chapter 5) that bind atoms to form molecules and molecules to form the animate and inanimate objects which make up the world we live in. These forms of work can only be sustained so long as energy is available.

Types of Energy

There are many forms of energy, including heat energy, chemical energy, electrical energy, magnetic energy and light energy. Of prime importance is the chemical energy which is obtained from fossil fuels such as coal and oil and the food we eat. Some of these will be covered in more detail in later sections.

Energy Conversions

Each type of energy can be converted to another type. For example, when coal is burned its chemical energy is converted to heat energy. A similar conversion occurs when food is eaten. Many industrial processes involve the conversion of energy from, for example, chemical energy to heat energy to electrical or mechanical energy. *Fig.* 2.1 shows the series of energy conversions involved in the production of the electric light which we all take so much for granted.

Every time energy is transformed, a certain amount will be dissipated and so become less useful. In a chain of energy transformations the amount of useful energy steadily declines. However, although energy can be converted from one form to another it can neither be created nor destroyed. There will *always* exist a constant cycle of energy conversions.

SOLAR ENERGY (the sun)

LIGHT ENERGY (photosynthesis of plants)

CHEMICAL ENERGY (coal)

HEAT ENERGY (coal-fired burners)

MECHANICAL ENERGY (steam turbine)

ELECTROMAGNETIC ENERGY (dynamo)

ELECTRICAL ENERGY (light bulb)

LIGHT ENERGY (activated light bulb)

Fig. 2.1 Series of energy conversions to activate a light bulb.

Kinetic and Potential Energy
Although there are many forms of energy (chemical, electrical etc.) each form can be manifested in only one of two modes, kinetic and potential. Thus there will be electrical potential energy and electrical kinetic energy, chemical potential energy and chemical kinetic energy etc. The words 'kinetic' and 'potential' thus indicate whether the type of energy under discussion is available to do work or is actually doing work.

Kinetic energy is the energy of motion. It is electrical and mechanical kinetic energy which makes machines and vehicles work. It is also the mode of energy which makes blood flow, and muscles move. The heat energy involved in the reactions of atoms is also in the form of kinetic energy.

Potential energy is stored energy. A coiled spring, a charged battery and a molecule of glucose all possess potential energy. It produces no change but has the power to cause

change when released under proper conditions. For example a glucose molecule has potential energy and when glucose is oxidized (Chapter 5) it will provide kinetic energy for living cells. Carbon and oxygen both contain chemical potential energy and at the appropriate temperature (the kindling temperature) they will unite and produce kinetic energy in the form of heat and light. Carbohydrates, lipids and proteins are all sources of chemical potential energy for the cell. This potential energy is liberated when large organic molecules are split into two or more smaller ones which together will contain less potential energy than the original molecule as some energy will be dissipated during the conversion in the form of heat. The potential chemical energy of food is eventually either used to do work or returned to the environment as heat.

Energy and Chemical Reactions
It may be easier to grasp the concept of work and energy in relation to physical activities than in relation to chemical reactions. It is not difficult to understand that the human body requires energy if it is to function (work). Neither is it difficult to understand that carbon and oxygen will combine to form carbon dioxide, but the fact that during the course of this reaction 100 000 calories are released for every 12 g of carbon used must not be overlooked. These calories can be used as a source of warmth or converted into other forms of energy, for instance steam or electricity. In order to convert the carbon dioxide back to carbon and oxygen, it would be necessary to supply exactly the same amount of energy as that which was released in the first reaction. The combination of carbon and oxygen is an energy-releasing or *exothermic* reaction. The reverse reaction, the breakdown of carbon dioxide into carbon and oxygen, is an energy-requiring or *endothermic* reaction.

Energy for Life Processes
The cells that make up the human body are constantly changing. Within a few days molecules have become 'old' and are broken down; at the same time new cells are being formed. Even apparently stable tissues such as bone and cartilage have been found to have quite a short life expectancy. The reproduction of

cells, contraction of muscles, transmission of messages through nerves and the secretion of hormones by specialized cells all represent work and so require energy.

Most cellular reactions require a source of energy and so are endothermic. The principal source of energy for the cell is glucose. This is broken down in a series of reactions, releasing only a small amount of energy each time. If the cell were to release a large amount of energy at one time it would be wasteful as much of the energy would be dissipated as heat, and more seriously, the cell would be unable to cope with this heat and would probably be destroyed.

Just as atomic power can be harnessed, controlled and released by atomic power stations in 'useful' quantities rather than in one vast atomic explosion, similarly the cell is able to convert glucose to carbon dioxide by a process involving almost 30 different reactions during each of which a small packet of energy is released. The cell is able to use this energy systematically to perform its many functions. To avoid waste all the energy released in the conversion of glucose to carbohydrate, and in other energy-releasing reactions, is used for the synthesis of adenosine triphosphate (ATP) and is thus conveniently stored (*see* Chapter 12).

Metabolism
The work done by the cell and the provision, production and utilization of the energy which makes this possible can be summed up in one word—*metabolism*. The process of metabolism includes all material and energy changes which occur and in its absence there will be no life. *Catabolism* and *anabolism* are its two components.

Protoplasm is constantly changing its form, producing heat and electrical energy (*see* Chapter 6) and undergoing chemical change (*see* Chapter 5). This activity is only possible if energy is available, and as protoplasm does not create energy it must derive it from carbohydrates, lipids and proteins (*see* Chapter 11). These are to be found in food but are also constituents of protoplasm. In order that this chemical potential energy (*see* Chapter 6) can

be utilized—as for example in muscle contraction—it must be released. It is this release of potential energy by protoplasm which is called catabolism.

When large organic molecules (*see* Chapter 12) split into two or more smaller molecules, the sum total of the potential energy contained in the new smaller molecules will be less than that which was contained in the original large molecule. The energy so liberated can be converted into other types of energy, for example mechanical energy for movement of whole or part of the body and for the transport of nutrients from one part of the body to another. It can also be converted to heat energy, which is necessary for the maintenance of body temperature. In mammals as much as 80 per cent of energy liberated in the protoplasm is converted to heat energy. Although catabolism occurs in all cells the degree of activity varies between different types of cell. The most active are those of muscle and liver whilst the least active are those found in connective tissue.

If the cell is to continue to exist, the molecules broken down during catabolism must be replaced. The processes involved in the synthesis or building up of the cell are collectively called anabolism. The first process, the supply of food, is followed by the breakdown or digestion of carbohydrates, lipids and proteins whose molecules are too large to pass into cells. This breakdown into molecules small enough to pass from the alimentary canal into the small blood vessels found in its wall is brought about by enzymes (*see* Chapter 12). Soluble nutrients can then be carried to all parts of the body to pass from the bloodstream into the intercellular fluid and so into the cells. Once in the cell nutrients can be used for various purposes such as the production of kinetic energy and the synthesis of monosaccharides, lipids, proteins etc. (*see* Chapter 12).

Metabolic Rates
An adult human at rest will utilize the minimum amount of energy necessary to maintain life. This is known as *basal metabolism*. It can be likened to the idling of a combustion engine

in a car that is not moving, when the minimum amount of energy (petrol) necessary to keep the engine running is being consumed. Movement of a resting body will stimulate an increase in catabolism, just as driving a car away will use more petrol.

Protoplasm possesses the fundamental characteristic of maintaining itself in a state of physiological equilibrium. Under normal conditions increased catabolism will be accompanied by—or quickly followed by—increased anabolism. Under abnormal conditions, for example during illness or when toxins are present, cells may be destroyed (catabolized) more rapidly than they can be replaced and this can lead to a situation where the amount of protoplasm is reduced to a degree where life can no longer be maintained. In childhood anabolism exceeds catabolism and growth arises either from an increase in the number of cells, or from an increase in the amount of protoplasm contained in existing cells.

The Source of Cellular Energy

Fig. 2.1 shows the sun to be the source of energy which, after a series of conversions, activates a light bulb. The sun is also the original source of the energy necessary to sustain human life. The potential chemical energy contained in food consumed is derived directly or indirectly from plants. Plants have the ability to synthesize simple substances such as water, carbon dioxide, nitrates, sulphates and phosphates into highly complex substances such as sugars, proteins, fats and starches. The energy needed for this conversion comes directly from the sun and the series of chemical reactions which brings about this change is known as 'photosynthesis'.

Animals are unable to perform this type of conversion and so take in the energy-rich material produced either directly by eating plants or indirectly by eating other animals which have eaten the plants. *Fig.* 2.2 shows the series of energy conversions leading to the support of human life processes.

Energy conversions performed by the living cell are 40 per cent efficient. This is much more economical than any mechanical (man-made) conversion method.

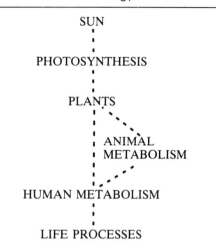

Fig. 2.2 The series of energy conversions involved in the support of life.

Motion

Energy is the capacity to do work and work is synonymous with change. In science work is always associated with movement of some kind, for example of machines, of leaves on a tree, of arms and legs, of nutrients and waste products into and out of living organism. Even a solid, inanimate object such as an oak table, which is apparently immobile, is made up of atoms (*see* Chapter 4) which are constantly in motion, vibrating (*see* Chapter 3), and of course all matter, including the living human organism, is made up of such atoms.

The movement of any object can only be described by referring to a previously fixed position, a point of origin (O). Objects can then be described as being a number (x) of units (miles, kilometres, centimetres) from that point. More exactly, the position of any object can be defined by its distance and direction from the point of origin. For instance, a geographical location will be defined as being 5 km west of a fixed position.

Before proceeding to a brief explanation of the laws of physics which govern the movement of all objects, it is necessary to differentiate between the terms speed, velocity, acceleration, mass and momentum.

Speed (s) is defined as the ratio of the distance covered by a moving body to the time taken. Average speed is the distance travelled divided by the time taken. Speed is a *scalar* quantity, that is it only has magnitude (size). It can refer to the movement of a body or to movement of substances, for example medicines, or radioactive isotopes (Chapter 5), through a body.

Velocity (v) is a measurement of both speed and a specified direction. To measure velocity the distance moved in a particular direction is divided by the time taken. A measurement which has magnitude (size) as well as direction is called a *vector* quantity. The voltage produced by the beating heart, which gives rise to the electrocardiogram, moves in a general direction from the centre of the chest to the left. This voltage has a vector quantity because it has both magnitude and direction.

Acceleration (a) is a measurement of how much the speed of a moving object has increased in a given time. In other words, it is a change in velocity per second.

Mass is concerned with what is commonly called weight. In everyday language 'weight' is used to indicate the measure of an object. Strictly speaking this is incorrect, as weight is a measure of the gravitational pull of the earth. Although the weight of any object varies little anywhere on earth, on the moon, where the earth's gravitational pull is only one-sixth of that on earth, the weight of any object will be only one-sixth of its value on earth. And in deep space, totally free of the gravitational pull of earth, all objects, including people, become weightless.

A more precise measure is therefore the mass of an object. This is a measure which depends on the number and size of the atoms contained in an object and is therefore a property that will not be affected by the earth's gravitational forces and so will remain constant on earth, on the moon or in deep space. The *density* of a substance is a measure of the amount of matter contained in a specific volume (e.g. 1 cm³ or 1 m³).

Momentum is another word that in everyday usage has different meanings. Moving objects, such as runaway vehicles, are said to be 'moving under their own momentum'. Political campaigns are sometimes described as 'gaining momentum'. In science, however, the word has a precise meaning: it is the product of mass multiplied by velocity. If the velocity of an object increases, then its momentum will increase. Because it depends on velocity, momentum is a vector quantity.

The Laws of Motion
In seventeenth century Italy, Galileo Galilei (1564–1642) began the study of moving bodies. This work was later furthered by Isaac Newton (1642–1727) in England. These studies showed that all forms of movement follow the same basic principles, which are summed up in Newton's three laws of motion.

The first law states that every body will continue in its state of rest or of motion at a constant speed in a straight line unless compelled by some external force to do otherwise. Here we must pause in our discussion to consider the word 'force'.

An object will not move unless something (a *force*) is pushing or pulling it. A force cannot be described in the same way that an object, such as a tree or an animal, can be described; it is only possible to state what a force can do.

When a body is acted upon by a force it will begin to move in a straight line. If the object is already moving the force may serve to alter its speed or direction or to cause it to stop moving. Force can therefore be defined as that which changes a body's state of rest or uniform motion in a straight line. That a push or a pull will cause an object to move, change direction or stop may be stating the obvious. Not so obvious perhaps is that an object, once set in motion, will continue to move in a straight line unless something stops it. The something that stops motion is *friction*.

Friction is itself a force and its effect will be appreciated when one considers the difficulties encountered when walking on a surface with little or no friction, such as a highly polished floor or a sheet of ice. Any solid object, including a human being, once set in motion (sliding) on ice will continue to move in a straight line until some friction prevents it or unless some other force changes its speed and direction. The smoother a surface the further the object will move before coming to a halt.

Types of Force
There are many types of force, including mechanical force (exerted by solid objects), elastic forces (exerted when solids are distorted), resistance forces (which oppose or prevent movement, for example air or wind resistance), electric forces (between electric charges, as in the atom), magnetic forces (which act on magnetic materials and on electric currents). But the type of force most generally encountered in everyday life is the force of gravity.

Gravity is well known as the force that pulls us towards the earth. What is perhaps not so readily appreciated is that gravitational forces exist between any two objects. For instance, two stones are not only attracted towards the earth, they are also attracted towards each other. Because stones are so small the gravitational force of attraction between them will not be noticed, although it can be measured by sensitive instruments. The strength of a force depends on the masses of the two objects and it will decrease as they get farther apart.

Centripetal force keeps a body moving in a circle (in orbit). It was once believed that planets were maintained in orbit by invisible spokes radiating from the sun. Since Isaac Newton we know that planets continue to move in their orbits because in the vacuum of outer space there is no opposing force (friction) to stop them. However, the gravitational attraction of the earth is needed to produce a continuous change of direction. Without this the 'orbiting' planet would continue in a straight line and would shoot off into deep space (until friction stopped it or until some other force changed its speed and direction).

Mechanics
If more than one force is acting on an object, and if the sum of the forces 'pulling' is equal to the sum of the forces 'pushing' (in other words, if the forces cancel each other out), then that object is said to be in a state of *equilibrium*. *Statics* is the study of objects in equilibrium and the science of statics is fundamental to many engineering feats, for instance bridge building. The study of systems which are not in equilibrium, or which are changing, is called *dyna-*

mics. The science of *mechanics* embraces both statics and dynamics.

The human body is itself a dynamic system because it is constantly changing, with cells being continually broken down and synthesized.

Pressure
In everyday language the word 'pressure' is often used to mean force, but for the scientist both have specific meanings and are not interchangeable. Consider these examples. When walking on snow, feet often sink but if skis or snow shoes are worn the likelihood of sinking is reduced. This is not because the force which caused the feet to sink has been reduced, but because the force has been spread over a greater area. The two ends of a drawing pin have very different surface areas. If this were not so then there would be a greater than 50:50 chance that the pin would end up in a thumb instead of in a piece of wood.

These examples indicate that *pressure* involves *area* as well as *force*. If a force is spread over a large area, then pressure is reduced. If force is spread over a small area, pressure is increased.

Air, which is a mixture of gases, exerts a pressure on earth and on all objects on earth. The average barometric pressure at sea level is 760 mmHg (millimetres of mercury) and this pressure is called 'standard atmospheric pressure' or 1 atmosphere. With increasing altitude atmospheric pressure decreases. Liquid exerts pressure in the same way, the pressure of a liquid increasing with depth. The unit of measurement of pressure is the newton (N).

An average-sized man, having a total surface area of 2 m², subject to normal atmospheric pressure, will have a total pressure acting on him in the region of 200 kN (kilo newtons). This is not normally noticeable because normal blood pressure is slightly higher than standard atmospheric pressure. At high altitudes, where air is less dense, atmospheric pressure decreases and so will be less than normal blood pressure and epistaxis may occur. Deep sea divers will be exposed to pressures greater than normal blood pressure and unless decompression is controlled, nitrogen bubbles form in the bloodstream causing decompression sickness, a condition commonly known as 'the bends'.

The second law of motion states that the momentum of a body is proportional to the applied force and takes place in the direction in which the force acts. The rate at which momentum is changed will depend on the value of the force applied. If a moving vehicle strikes a solid object, deceleration will be rapid and the velocity of the moving vehicle quickly reduced to zero. When two objects such as a heavy laden lorry and a light car are acted upon by the same degree of force for the same period of time, the small object will build up a higher velocity (speed and direction) than the larger one, but the momentum they gain will be the same in both cases.

The third law of motion states that whenever a force acts on a body, an equal but opposite force acts on some other body. In other words, to every action there is an equal and opposite reaction.

When a force acts there are always two objects involved. For instance, a person lean-ing against a tree will exert a force on the tree, but the tree will also exert a force on the person and these forces will be equal in strength but opposite in direction. The action and reaction associated with firing a gun will be more obvious. When a gun is fired, the action of the bullet passing down the barrel will be accompanied by the equal backward (opposite) reaction of the recoil of the gun. The same principle applies to the firing of a rocket. The burning of fuel produces a high velocity blast of gas and it is the reaction to the force of the gas which causes the body of the rocket to move in the opposite direction.

When two bodies collide they will exert the same degree of force on each other. The total momentum of the two will be unaltered by the collision and this is known as the *principle of conservation of momentum*. The principle applies equally to collisions between solid bodies and to explosions (as in the burning of rocket fuel).

Newton's laws of motion are applicable to all moving objects regardless of size. They can be applied to human beings and machines, planets and moons in orbit and to molecules of gases.

3

Vibrations and waves

All movement discussed so far has involved the movement of a body from one point (A) to another point (B). There are some things, however, which are constantly moving yet never actually get anywhere. The atoms in a solid for instance, including those which make up the living body, are constantly moving yet they do not alter their mean position relative to each other. If they did then there would be no 'solid' objects as we know them!

Such movement is known as *vibration* and vibrating objects are commonplace. Sounds, for instance, are produced mainly by vibrations of stretched strings or by vibrations of air in pipes. The human body is itself a vibrating system and it can also be affected by external vibrations. The moving pendulum in a clock, the loaded spring and the ball in a cylinder are other examples of vibrating objects (*see Fig.* 3.1).

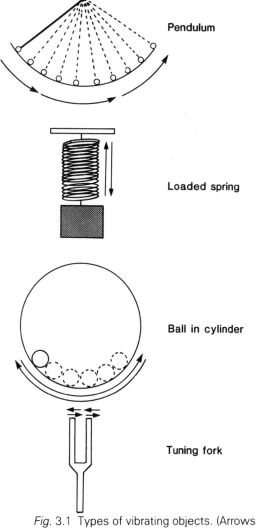

Features of Vibrations
Despite the diversity of types of vibrating objects, there are a number of common features and similar movements which can be observed, and a number of differences which can be noted, in each case.
- Movement is backwards and forwards between two extreme points.
- The movement repeats itself exactly for a number of times then gradually gets less and less and eventually stops.
- Speed of movement is *not* constant throughout; there are periods of acceleration and retardation.

Fig. 3.1 Types of vibrating objects. (Arrows indicate direction of movement.)

- In any particular system a vibration takes the same length of time, irrespective of the size of the movement.
- All systems *do not* have the same vibration time.
- The time taken for vibrations to die away will be different in different systems.

The Cycle

A complete vibration (or oscillation) is called a *cycle* and is one complete to and fro movement. For example, where A is the central point and B and C the extremes of movement, a complete cycle would be the movement from A–B–A–C and back to A (*see Fig.* 3.2).

Amplitude

The distance between the centre point and the extreme point on either side is a measure of the size, or *amplitude*, of the vibration. Where A is the centre point and B and C the extremes of movement, the amplitude is the distance between A and B or between A and C (*see Fig.* 3.3).

Periodic Time

The time taken for a particular vibration to complete one cycle is called the *periodic time*. To determine this it is usual to measure the time taken to complete ten or more cycles when the average time can be found by

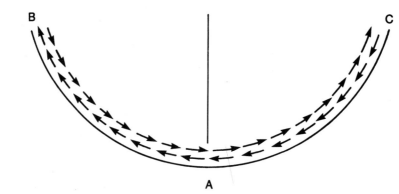

Fig. 3.2 One complete cycle of a vibration.

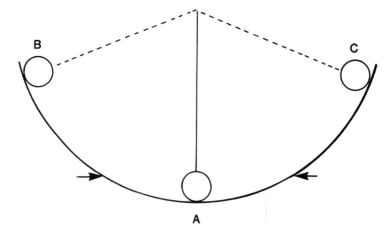

Fig. 3.3 A measurement of amplitude, A–B or A–C.

dividing the time taken by the number of vibrations.

Frequency
It is often more convenient to use a measure of *frequency* rather than one of periodic time. Frequency is a measure of the number of cycles which occur in one second. The unit of frequency is the hertz (Hz).

Resonance
All objects have a frequency at which they will vibrate if left free to do so. For instance, if a child's swing is set in motion or a diving board is bent they will vibrate at their natural frequencies if left to move freely. Any extra force (energy) which is applied to coincide with the natural frequency will cause the object to vibrate with very large amplitude; for instance, pushing a swing upwards as it begins its upward motion. This effect is called *resonance*. A glass tumbler shattered by an opera singer is another example; the note sung, being equal to the natural frequency of the glass, will create vibrations of sufficient amplitude to shatter the glass.

Energy and Vibration
Every action and reaction involves an exchange of energy (*see* Chapter 2), and vibrating objects are no exception. Any object or system will require an input of energy, for example electrical or mechanical, to set it in motion. Once in motion, the velocity (speed and direction) of the vibrating object will be changing throughout the movement. This will involve alternating conversions between kinetic and potential energy. Some energy will be dissipated, so unless more energy is added, the vibrations will eventually stop. *Fig.* 3.4 shows how kinetic energy and potential energy conversions occur alternately.

Vibrations and Health
Vibration is a recognized occupational hazard. Inevitably, increasing mechanization has increased sources of vibration. In all forms of transport, land, sea and air, vibrations will be transmitted through the structure of the vehicle (car, ship, aeroplane) to the individual. Heavy machinery, such as forges and compressors, is also a source of body vibration and hand-held tools, such as chain saws, are sources of localized vibration.

The effects of external vibration on humans depend on several factors including the frequency and amplitude of the vibration, duration of exposure and, in the case of whole body exposure, direction of the vibration. In the human body three axes of vibration, X, Y, and Z, are normally identified (*see Fig.* 3.5). These are:
- Horizontal vibration from the front to the back of the chest (X).

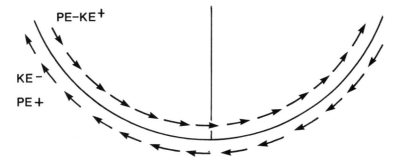

Potential energy increasing, kinetic energy decreasing

PE–KE+

KE–
PE+

Potential energy decreasing, kinetic energy increasing

Fig. 3.4 Alternate conversions of kinetic and potential energy.

- Horizontal vibration from shoulder to shoulder (Y).
- Vertical vibration through the central axis of a person sitting or standing (Z).

Effects of Vibration on Living Tissue

The human body will absorb most vibratory energy that is applied to it between 0·5 and 20 Hz and so is most sensitive to vibrations within this range. The human body is itself a vibrating system and is therefore subject to resonance. Any applied vibration which coincides with the natural frequencies of the body will therefore create vibrations of greater amplitude. The natural frequencies of some parts of the human body are shown in Table 3.1.

Animal studies have shown that tissue damage will occur at natural frequencies for specific limbs or organs. In humans no laboratory studies have been possible, and only humans who have been accidentally affected

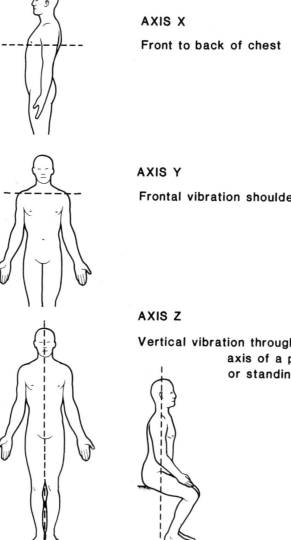

AXIS X

Front to back of chest

AXIS Y

Frontal vibration shoulder to shoulder

AXIS Z

Vertical vibration through the central axis of a person sitting or standing.

Fig. 3.5 The three axes of vibration of the human body.

can be observed. Whole body vibration is known to be a cause of discomfort and loss of efficiency. Motion sickness, blurred vision and impaired visual acuity can also occur. It has been suggested that a fatal ruptured aorta in a helicopter pilot was due to exposure to extreme vibration when his craft lost its blades (Zenz, 1975). Localized vibration occurs when hand-held tools are used and this can result in vibration-induced white finger (Reynaud's phenomenon).

Table 3.1 Natural frequencies in the human body

Body part	Natural frequency (Hz)
Hand	30–40
Lower jaw	100–200
Head	20–30
Eyeball	60–90

Waves

Many vibrating objects produce *waves* that radiate from them, for example light and sound waves. A wave allows energy to be transferred from one point to another either through a vacuum, as in the case of light, or through a medium, as with sound. Although there are many types of wave, the nature and properties of all waves are the same.

If a long spring is placed on a flat surface and one end is shaken at right-angles to its length, then a wave motion will be set up and the wave will be moving at right-angles to the length of the spring. This is termed a *transverse wave*. Light waves are examples of transverse waves (*see Fig.* 3.6).

If the spring is shaken in the direction of the length of the spring, then a concertina effect occurs. The wave travels along the length of the spring. This is called a *longitudinal* wave. Sound waves are an example of longitudinal waves (*see Fig.* 3.6).

Definitions

Amplitude

Amplitude (*a*) is the maximum displacement of the wave from zero (or starting) position. The unit of amplitude is the metre (m) (*see Fig.* 3.7).

Wavelength

Wavelength (λ) is the distance between corresponding points on two successive waves. The unit of measurement is the metre (m) (*see Fig.* 3.7).

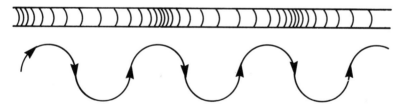

Fig. 3.6 Types of wave formation. *a*, Transverse waves—areas of compression and rarefaction in a spring; *b*, longitudinal waves.

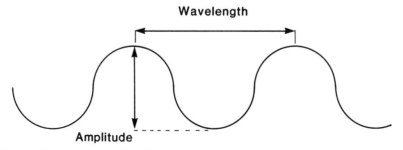

Fig. 3.7 Amplitude and wavelength.

Frequency

The number of waves produced per second is known as the *frequency* (*f*).

Speed

The length of each wave (λ) multiplied by the number of waves per second (*f*) will give the *speed* (*v*) or velocity of the wave motion. Thus

$$v = f\lambda$$

Properties of Waves

Reflection

When any wave reaches a barrier it will be reflected. The whispering gallery of St Paul's Cathedral in London is one example of the reflection of sound waves. (For discussion of sound waves *see* p.20.) In this circular chamber sound waves are repeatedly bounced or reflected off the walls so that a person whispering at one end can be clearly heard at the other. Echoes are the product of sound reflected from a hard surface such as a cliff or a wall.

Sound travels at about 33 metres per second (33 ms^{-1}) so the reflected sound wave must travel a distance of at least 33 m for the echo to be heard separately from the original sound. Thus, if the wall or cliff is less than 17 m distant the echo follows so quickly that it cannot be distinguished from the original sound and the impression gained is that the sound is prolonged. This is known as *reverberation* and is particularly noticeable in large buildings such as cathedrals. In St Paul's Cathedral for instance, the sound of the organ does not fade away for about 6 seconds after the organist has stopped playing.

Sources of light, such as the sun, stars and electric lamps, can be seen when the light they produce reaches the eyes. However, most objects can only be seen when light bounces (is reflected) off the surface of an object. An object that reflects no light appears to be black whilst an object that reflects all of the light appears the same colour as the light source, for instance something which reflects all of the white light reaching it from the sun appears white.

A sheet of white paper and a highly polished silvery surface such as a mirror, will reflect all of the light that falls on them. The different appearance of these two objects occurs because of the difference in the finish of the two surfaces. A mirror is very smooth and so will reflect all light rays reaching it from a specific source in one direction only, this is known as *regular reflection*. From the relatively rough surface of paper there will be irregular scattering of reflected light rays and this is known as *diffuse reflection* (*see* Fig. 3.8).

One application of reflected light is the endoscope, which is used for examining those parts of the body which the eyes cannot reach. It consists of a bundle of solid glass fibres which carry light around corners by a series of internal reflections. The image transmitted is composed of light and dark dots, each dot being made by a separate fibre. Optical fibres are also extensively used in the communications industry. Laser light can be used to convey information, for example telephone conversations, computer data, television pictures. An optical fibre has the same capacity as a copper cable which is ten times thicker. Not only are optical fibres smaller, they are also cheaper than metals such as copper which are becoming increasingly scarce and expensive.

Refraction

When a wave crosses a boundary of two different media it is bent or *refracted*. This effect can be seen by dipping a pencil or ruler into a glass of water. That part which is under the water will appear to be bent.

Refraction occurs because when the density of a medium changes the velocity (speed and direction) changes also. This is why sound is easier to hear at night. The density of air, which is a mixture of gases, is altered by changes in temperature. When passing through layers of air of different temperatures sound waves will be refracted. At night, when the air near the ground is cool, sound waves will be bent (refracted) downwards and sound will be heard more easily. On a hot day sound waves will be refracted upwards towards cooler air, making hearing more difficult.

The speed of light in a vacuum is 3×10^8 (300 000 000) metres per second, but in transparent materials it travels more slowly and this change in speed is accompanied by refraction.

The same laws of refraction apply when

light travels in the opposite direction, that is from the denser transparent medium to air. This is known as the principle of *reversibility of light*. It means simply that if two rays of light are sent in exactly the same direction they will both follow the same path. (*See Fig.* 3.9.)

The extent of bending (refraction) which occurs depends on both the media which the light wave is leaving and that which it is entering. This is indicated by the *refractive index* or strictly speaking the *relative* refractive index. For convenience, all transparent mater-

ials are given a value known as the *absolute refractive index* and this indicates the amount of bending that would occur if a ray of light passed from a vacuum into a transparent medium. In fact, the degree of refraction of light passing from a vacuum is almost the same as that which occurs when it passes from air into the same medium. In practice it is assumed that light is entering the medium from air and the word 'absolute' is often omitted. *Table* 3.2 lists the absolute index of some familiar materials.

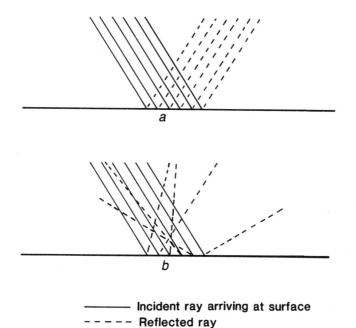

——— **Incident ray arriving at surface**

– – – – – **Reflected ray**

Fig. 3.8 The reflection of light. *a*, Regular reflection of light from smooth (mirror) surface; *b*, diffuse reflection of light from rough (paper) surface.

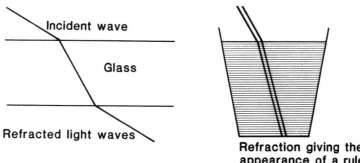

Incident wave

Glass

Refracted light waves

Refraction giving the appearance of a ruler bending in water

Fig. 3.9 The refraction of light.

Table 3.2 Absolute refractive index of various materials

Medium	Absolute refractive index
Glass	1.48–1.96 (according to composition)
Perspex	1.5
Water	1.33
Ice	1.3
Diamond	2.4

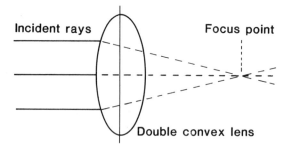

Fig. 3.11 Light passing through a double convex lens.

White light consists of seven different colours, each having a different wavelength. A white light passing through a glass prism, which is a denser medium than air, will split into a *spectrum*, a series of parallel beams of light of different colours. These are familiar as the colours of the rainbow, red, orange, yellow, green, blue, indigo and violet, which are seen when a beam of light is dispersed through water (rain). This dispersion of colours occurs because the differences in wavelength of the various colours cause them to be refracted at different angles (*see Fig.* 3.10). The change of the colours which make up white light is gradual, there are no sudden changes and no gaps. Such a spectrum is described as a *continuous spectrum*.

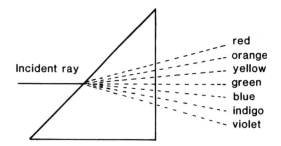

Fig. 3.10 The refraction of white light in a prism.

Glass lenses, like the lens of the human eye, work by refraction. Light rays passing through are refracted and, depending on the shape of the lens, will emerge travelling in a different direction. *Fig.* 3.11 shows how parallel rays of light bend to meet at a single focus point after passing through a double convex lens.

Diffraction

Consider what happens when straight waves travel towards two vertical barriers with an opening between them. If the opening is wide in comparison to the length of the waves then they will pass through in parallel straight lines. However, should the opening be about the same size as the wavelength, then after passing through the opening the waves will spread out in all directions. This is called *diffraction*.

It is diffraction which causes sound waves to spread around corners and is the reason why sounds can be heard even though a solid barrier exists between the source and the receiver. For example, the opening of a doorway 1 metre wide is similar in size to the wavelength of many sounds and these will be diffracted. However, the range of sounds is vast, from 20 cm to 10 m, so soundwaves of shorter wavelengths, that is those which produce high-pitched sounds, will not be diffracted so much. This is why high-pitched sounds tend to be more directional than the low-pitched sounds of longer wavelength. From a loudspeaker, high pitched sounds are best heard from in front, rather than at the side or behind a speaker.

Diffraction also allows light to travel around corners where light, which travels in a straight line, should not normally go. However, when a beam of light passes through a large gap diffraction will be negligible. The wavelength of visible light lies between 4×10^{-7} and $7 \cdot 7 \times 10^{-7}$ m, so it is only when light passes through a very narrow slit that diffraction can be observed (*see Fig.* 3.12).

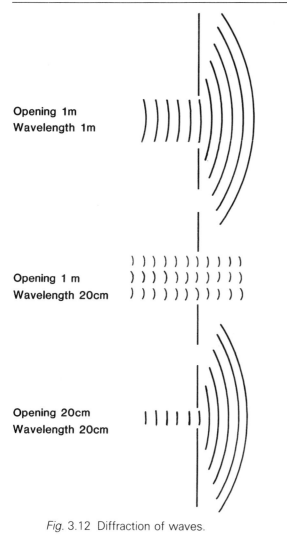

Opening 1m
Wavelength 1m

Opening 1 m
Wavelength 20cm

Opening 20cm
Wavelength 20cm

Fig. 3.12 Diffraction of waves.

Interference

When waves from separate sources but of the same frequency meet there will be areas where the two waves overlap. In some places the disturbance at these points of overlap will be practically zero, whilst at others the disturbance will be about twice that which would have resulted from one wave alone. This is because when one wave is superimposed on another, the amplitude at any point will be the sum of the amplitude of the two waves. This is called *interference*. If the peaks and troughs of the two waves correspond exactly, that is when they are in phase, they will reinforce each

other so that the actual displacement (amplitude) will be greater than that of each wave taken separately. If the peaks and troughs of the two waves do not correspond then cancellation will occur (*see* Fig. 3.13).

Constructive interference of sound waves produces regions of louder sound, whilst *destructive* interference produces regions of quiet. Interference between light waves can also be constructive, producing more light, but in some places where they overlap destructive interference results in darkness.

Destructive interference

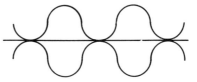

Constructive interference

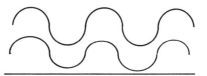

Constructive

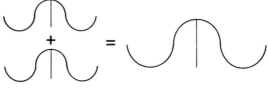

Destructive

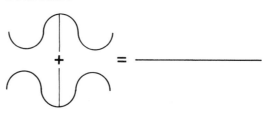

Fig. 3.13 Interference of waves.

Sound Waves

Whenever a fluctuating disturbance is produced in a medium such as air, water, metal or lastic, the disturbance will spread out from the source and there will be a transfer of momentum from one molecule to the next. Such disturbances are known as sound waves. Sound waves will not travel in a vacuum.

The speed at which the disturbance, or sound, travels is determined by the properties of the medium (density, temperature). In air at a temperature of 20 °C sound travels at a velocity of about 330 metres per second (330 ms^{-1}); this is much slower than the velocity of light ($3 \times 10^8 \text{ ms}^{-1}$) and accounts for the delay between the sighting of a flash of lightning and the hearing of the sound wave (thunder) which it produces. Sound waves are in fact pressure disturbances and because the range of sound pressures is so wide, it is more convenient to measure noise on a logarithmic scale (*see* Appendix 1) called the decibel scale (*see* Appendix 3).

The tone or pitch of sound is determined by its frequency, which is measured in hertz (Hz) (*see* Appendix 3). Middle C on the music scale is 256 Hz whilst the Greenwich time signal is 1000 Hz. Noise rarely consists of a single tone though, so when noise is measured it is important to measure the whole frequency spectrum of any particular noise source.

Audible sound falls between frequencies 20–16 000 Hz but the range of frequencies extends both above and below these normal limits of human hearing.

Noise at frequencies below 20 Hz is produced by a wide range of machines such as diesel engines and poorly designed ventilation systems. Frequencies at about 7 Hz may interfere with the alpha rhythms of the biocircuits of the brain. Frequencies between 2 Hz and 5 Hz may give rise to resonance, and resonance of internal organs can cause subjective sensations. Noise at such lower frequencies is called *infrasound*.

High frequency sounds—*ultrasound*—are inaudible to the human ear. Bats use such sounds to locate obstacles in the dark. During World War II the same method was used to detect submarines underwater.

A high frequency sound can be reflected off any object and a complete picture of that object can be built up from the pattern of reflections. In the 1950s this technique was introduced into medicine to study the unborn fetus. Today ultrasound is commonly used in obstetrics to determine the size and position of the fetus. It is also used for the diagnosis of diseases of the heart, lungs and liver.

Electromagnetic Waves

As early as 1690 Christian Huygens (1629–95) had suggested that light could travel in waves. But Isaac Newton (1642–1727) applied his laws of motion to light and was led to suggest that light travels in small particles, which he called 'corpuscles'. Although Newton's theory accounted for reflection and refraction, it did not explain the properties of diffraction and interference, whereas all of the properties of light could be explained by regarding light as travelling in waves. In 1801 the English physicist and physician Thomas Young (1773–1829) revived the wave theory of light. In experiments he found that light of the same frequency which was diffracted (spread out) after passing through two pin holes produced a pattern of light and dark bands on a screen placed in the path of the light. The light bands corresponded to areas of *constructive* interference and the dark bands to areas of *destructive* interference. In this way Young produced strong evidence in support of the wave theory of light.

At the beginning of this century, the German physicist Max Planck (1858–1947) introduced his now famous *quantum theory*. He concluded that energy (light) does not flow continuously from hot bodies but is emitted in small packets called 'quanta' or 'photons', the amount of energy carried by a photon depending on the wavelength, or frequency, of the emission. Such energy can be considered as particles that exist as waves. It seems therefore that neither Newton nor Huygens was either totally right or totally wrong.

In 1845 Michael Faraday showed that light waves passing through a medium were affected by magnetic fields. (At this time the connection between electricity and magnetism was recognized; *see* Chapter 6). Subsequently James Clerk Maxwell suggested that an oscillating electric current should be capable of radiating energy in the form of electromagnetic waves. In 1888 Heinrich Hertz (1857–94) showed that electromagnetic waves could be produced by means of an oscillating electric spark and that the waves produced underwent reflection, refraction and diffraction. They were in fact like light waves, but of a different wavelength, thus suggesting that light waves themselves were electromagnetic, a belief which has subsequently been confirmed.

It was the work of Hertz which led to the development by Marconi and others of the use of electromagnetic waves for radio communication.

A whole range of electromagnetic waves reach earth from the sun and outer space and these conform to the behaviour properties of all waves. Because all electromagnetic waves travel at the same speed in a vacuum (3×10^8 ms^{-1}) the wavelength of any frequency can readily be calculated using the equation connecting wavelength, frequency and velocity ($v = f\lambda$). When dealing with electromagnetic waves, particularly when in a vacuum, velocity is normally represented by the symbol c.

The Electromagnetic Spectrum (Appendix 2)

The electromagnetic spectrum is divided into ranges which are referred to as 'bands'. The name assigned to a band may refer to the source of the radiation or its application. Like the spectrum of colours in white light, the electromagnetic spectrum is continuous. Although there are different types of radiation, there are no gaps, no frequencies which do not exist and no sharp boundaries between one type of radiation and another. There is in fact often a large overlap in boundaries. A wavelength of 1 mm for instance can be either infrared or microwave.

Light waves fall into the middle of the spectrum and have wavelengths ranging from 0.4 to 0.7 micrometres (μm). The longest wavelengths belong to radio waves, the shortest to gamma and X-rays.

All electromagnetic waves originate in energy changes which can involve the nuclei or electronic structure of atoms. For instance, gamma rays are emitted by decaying atomic nuclei and X-rays are generated when high speed electrons penetrate an atom to reach its inner electrons or its nucleus (*see* Chapter 4).

Wavelengths can therefore be separated in terms of energy. Ultraviolet radiation (wavelengths shorter than visible violet light) causes sunburn, whereas infrared (wavelengths longer than red visible light) only warms the skin. All parts of the spectrum transfer energy from a source to a receiver, the energy travelling in the form of an oscillating electric and magnetic field.

Special Properties

Electromagnetic waves exhibit some common properties but there are also some special properties typical of particular wavelengths.

Gamma rays originate in the nucleus of radioactive atoms (*see* Chapter 4) and cosmic rays. They are very penetrating photons of dangerously high energy. In medicine they are used in the treatment of cancers and can also be used for sterilization, for example of syringes and instruments. In some countries food is sterilized by gamma irradiation.

The gamma camera can detect rays from radionuclides and a clear picture of both bones and soft tissues can be obtained. The development of the gamma camera has reduced the use of earlier X-ray techniques. In industry gamma rays are used in non-destructive testing of metals.

X-rays have the same dangerous penetrating power as gamma rays (both are 'ionizing radiations', *see* Chapter 4). The medical radiological uses of X-rays are well known. They are also used for non-destructive testing in industry and for the study of the structure of solids (X-ray crystallography).

Ultraviolet waves originate in the sun and very hot objects. Ultraviolet radiation can damage living tissue causing severe burns and it is particularly dangerous to the eyes, which must always be protected. It can kill living organisms and is used in the food and catering industries to destroy insects. Arc welding is a well-known source of ultraviolet radiation in industry. Ultraviolet lamps are used for the treatment of some skin conditions.

Infrared waves originate in the sun and warm objects, including human beings. All objects emit and absorb infrared radiation simultaneously. If more is absorbed than emitted the temperature of the object increases and vice versa. Infrared is invisible heat energy; the red glow of a fire is *not* due to infrared radiation. The hottest part of an object contains and emits infrared radiation of higher frequency, a fact which enables photographs to be taken at night using special photographic film. Photographs can also be taken from space which reveal buildings, people, missile sites etc. by virtue of their different temperatures.

Radio waves cover a wide range of wavelengths from one centimetre to hundreds of kilometres. Microwaves are the shortest radio waves and there is considerable overlap between these and infrared waves. Both provide energy for cooking. Microwaves are also used in radio, telephone and radar systems for communication.

Television pictures are transmitted via an aerial by ultra high frequency (UHF) radio waves. Very high frequency (VHF) waves, which typically have wavelengths of 3 m provide the radio waves received by direct transmission from transmitter to receiver over short distances.

Common Properties

Electromagnetic waves carry no electrical charge. They all transfer energy from one place to another and can be both absorbed and emitted by matter. They obey the laws of reflection, refraction and diffraction. They need no medium to travel through and all travel at the same speed (the speed of light, i.e. 3×10^8 m^{-1}).

Ionizing Radiations (see also Chapter 4)

All radiation can be dangerous under certain conditions. For example, infrared and microwaves can damage living tissue. Radiations which possess energy greater than that of ultraviolet radiation have the power to dislodge electrons from the atoms with which they interact. Thus the atoms, by losing one or more of their orbiting electrons, become ions or have been 'ionized'. Any radiation which has the power to do this is called an *ionizing radiation*.

In high enough doses such radiation can be harmful to living cells. Chemical changes occur almost immediately and biological changes, depending on dosage, can occur from seconds to decades after exposure. In the healthy human cell death and renewal (metabolism, *see* Chapter 2) is a normal on-going process. Radiation becomes harmful when it results in damage to DNA or in the death of so many cells that the body can no longer function efficiently.

The properties of ionizing radiations can be used to beneficial effect in the treatment of disease, in particular the treatment of cancer. *Radiotherapy* includes selective irradiation with X-rays and other ionizations as well as the ingestion or implantation of radioisotopes.

Reference

Zenz, Carl *Occupational Medicine*. Chicago, Year Book, 1975.

4

Elements and atoms

The universe and all material things in it are made up of basic particles called *atoms*. The Greek philosopher Democritus (460–370 BC) was amongst the first to suggest all matter to be composed of indestructible and indivisible particles moving about in space. He called these particles *atoma* meaning 'indivisible'. Democritus asserted that substances differed in density and this difference was dependent on the ratio of particles to spaces, less dense substances having more open spaces. This idea was largely ignored for 2000 years: not only was there no evidence to support it, but Aristotle (384-322 BC), probably the most influential of the Greek philosophers, rejected the idea. He lent his support to the theory of matter being composed of just four elements— earth (solid), water (liquid), air (gas) and fire (an intangible element)—believing all material things to be a combination of these elements in varying proportions. Aristotle's support of this theory may well have led to its continued dominance throughout the Middle Ages.

Dalton's Atomic Theory
The concept of 'indestructible and indivisible particles' came to be widely accepted only after the chemist John Dalton (1766–1844) commenced work on his atomic theory in 1803. Dalton proposed all matter to be composed of elements that can neither be created nor destroyed. He believed all atoms of the same element to be alike but atoms of different elements to have different weights. He devised a scale of 'atomic weights' by selecting a standard element—he chose oxygen—and arbitrarily assigning to it a value—he chose 8.

He then measured the weights of other elements which combined with a given amount of oxygen. (He assumed, wrongly it transpired, that one atom of oxygen would combine with one atom of another element.) With this information he calculated the weights of elements: for example

7·0 g of oxygen combines with 83·0 g of mercury

so

8·0 g of oxygen will combine with $83 \times 8/7 = 95\cdot0$ g of mercury

therefore

if the atomic weight of oxygen is 8, the atomic weight of mercury is 95.

Dalton's theory was not universally accepted until the latter end of the nineteenth century by which time 58 elements had been identified. The principle of arbitrarily assigning a weight to a particular element and measuring the weights of other elements relative to this is still applied today. The element of choice now is carbon-12, which is defined as having a mass (weight) of 12 atomic mass units (amu) and the masses of other elements are relevant to this standard. Any trace of impurity will affect the accuracy of the measurement and methods of purification can alter the relative proportions of the elements present in the sample. Technology has now provided the mass spectrometer, however, as the means of determining relative atomic masses. This not only requires smaller samples, but impurities do not matter.

Families of Elements
It was recognized that some elements,

although differing in atomic weight (mass), showed similar properties. For instance the halogen (salt forming) elements—chlorine, bromine, iodine—and the alkali metals—lithium, sodium, potassium. In 1869 the Russian scientist Mendeleev arranged all known elements in order of atomic weight so that different 'families' were grouped together. He was not deterred by the presence of elements which, according to their calculated weight, did not fit into the plan. He assumed, correctly, that the weight was wrong. Neither did gaps in the table worry him, for he believed that these would subsequently be filled by elements that were yet to be discovered. As his idea won acceptance chemists began actively (and successfully) to search for the missing elements. There are now 105 elements known to man. Of these 90 are naturally occurring, the remainder have been created in laboratories as the result of nuclear reactions.

The Relative Abundance of Elements
All elements do not exist in similar proportions. For instance 99 per cent of the whole universe consists of only two elements, hydrogen and helium, a large percentage of these two elements being in outer space. Of the remaining 1 per cent, oxygen is the most abundant. Ninety-nine per cent of the substances occurring on the earth and in the earth's atmosphere are made up of only nine elements. The estimated percentage composition of these nine is shown in *Table* 4.1. The most important of the elements that make up the human body are shown in *Table* 4.2.

Table 4.1 Estimated percentage composition of the nine major elements occurring on earth and in the earth's atmosphere

Element	%
Oxygen	49·2
Silicon	25·7
Aluminium	7·5
Iron	4·7
Calcium	3·4
Sodium	2·8
Potassium	2·6
Magnesium	1·9
Hydrogen	0·9

Table 4.2 The most important elements within the human body

Element	%
Oxygen	65
Carbon	18
Hydrogen	10
Nitrogen	3
Calcium	2
Phosphorus	1·1
Chlorine	0·15
Potassium	0·35
Sodium	0·15
Sulphur	0·25
Magnesium	
Iron	
Copper	
Manganese	traces
Zinc	
Cobalt	
Iodine	

The Basic Ingredients
Elements are the basic ingredients of all substances. Atoms of the same element may join together to produce a pure substance and atoms of two or more different elements may join to form *compounds*. This building of compounds from basic elements is known as *synthesis*. Manufactured goods ranging from man-made fibres to medicinal compounds are often described as 'synthetic'. The breaking down of compounds into basic elements is known as *analysis*.

Atoms
The belief that atoms are indivisible was proved wrong when the first sub-atomic particle was discovered by J. J. Thompson (1856–1940) in 1897. This particle was the negatively charged electron. In 1911 Ernest Rutherford (1871–1937) demonstrated that the atom is composed of a *nucleus*—containing the mass of the atom—surrounded by *electrons*. The nucleus contains protons and neutrons (known collectively as *nucleons*). Protons carry a positive electrical charge while neutrons, as the name implies, carry no electrical charge (*see* Chapter 5). Because the atom could no longer

be said to be indivisible, the original definition no longer held true. Now an atom is defined as the smallest part of an element which can take part in a chemical reaction. It cannot be further divided without changing the element's identity.

If all matter is made up of small particles, why is it that so much of the world appears to be solid and indivisible? What is it that joins atoms together so effectively that they form structures such as living creatures, plants and rocks? To answer these questions we need first to look more closely at the structure of the atom.

The Structure of the Atom

Atoms are composed of negatively charged electrons, positively charged protons and neutrons which have no charge. The negative charge of the electron is equal in strength, although opposite in charge, to the positive charge of the proton.

Protons and neutrons are contained in a nucleus which has a diameter of approximately 10^{-15} m. Electrons form a cloud around the nucleus extending to a radius of about 10^{-10} m. These sub-atomic particles are held together by two different types of force. The nuclear force which holds the nucleons in the nucleus, and the electromagnetic force which holds the electrons in orbit around the nucleus.

Because the number of negatively charged electrons is equal to the number of positively charged protons, the atom remains neutral. The number of electrons orbiting the nucleus (or the number of protons in the nucleus, which is the same) is known as the atomic number (Z) and this ranges from 1 (hydrogen) to 105 (hahnium). Usually the nucleus contains the same number of neutrons as protons. However the ratio of neutrons to protons increases slowly as the atomic number, and therefore the number of protons, increases. The simplest atom is the hydrogen atom which is composed of one electron and one proton only. It is the only atom which does not possess a neutron (*see Fig.* 4.1).

The atom has been likened to a solar system because both have a mass at the centre—the sun or the nucleus—which is surrounded by other bodies—planets or electrons. But this anology is not quite accurate because electrons orbit the nucleus so fast—thousands of millions of times in a millionth of a second—that no method of measurement can be devised to determine where they are at any given time. The position of the planets surrounding the sun can, on the other hand, easily be established. The atom is more correctly described as a dense nucleus surrounded by a cloud of electrical charge formed by the orbiting electrons. This is known as the *cloud of probability*. In its normal state the simplest atom, hydrogen, will assume a spherical shape (*see Fig.* 4.2). If the atom is excited, that is if it is supplied with more energy, the electron cloud will become larger and possibly dumbbell shaped (*see Fig.* 4.3). In more complex atoms, such as carbon, which has six electrons, the orbiting electrons are arranged in spherical layers or shells (*see Fig.* 4.4).

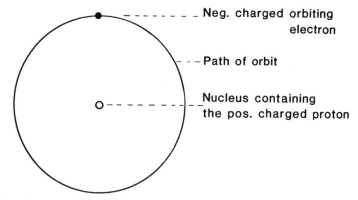

Fig. 4.1 The structure of the hydrogen atom.

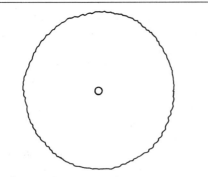

Fig. 4.2 The shape of the hydrogen atom in its normal (unexcited) state.

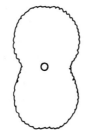

Fig. 4.3 The shape of the excited hydrogen atom.

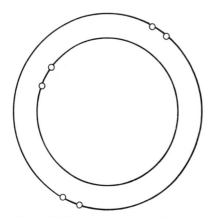

Fig. 4.4 The arrangement of electrons in a carbon atom.

Isotopes and Nuclides

Atoms of specific elements will often be referred to as *isotopes* or *nuclides*.

Atoms of the same element may differ in atomic mass because although their nuclei contain the same number of protons they may contain different numbers of neutrons. Such atoms are called *isotopes* of the element. Hydrogen for example has three isotopes in which the nucleus contains two, one or no neutrons respectively. The isotopes of hydrogen have been given specific names, tritium, deuterium and prontium (*see Table* 4.3). No other element has been awarded this distinction. Isotopes are identified by their atomic number and mass number and are usually referred to by the name of the element and the number of neutrons in the nucleus, for example carbon-12, carbon-13, carbon-14 (*see* Appendix 6).

Table 4.3 The composition of isotopes of hydrogen

Isotope	Protons	Neutrons	Electrons
Tritium	1	2	1
Deuterium	1	1	1
Prontium	1	0	1

The word nuclide refers to the nucleus of a specific isotope and is identified by its atomic number, mass number *and* its energy state (*see* Chapter 5). Atoms undergoing radioactive decay are often referred to as nuclides.

NB: An isotope refers to a type of atom whilst a nuclide refers to its nucleus.

Ions

Electrons can break free from one type of material and adhere to another. When an electron breaks free from its atom the negative charge of the electrons will no longer equal the positive charge of the protons and so the atom will contain a positive charge. Similarly, when an electron adheres to another atom, that atom will acquire a negative charge. Any such electrically charged atom—or group of atoms—is called an *ion*. Positively charged ions are called *cations*; they have fewer electrons than necessary for the atom to remain neutral. Negative ions, which are called *anions*, have more.

Radioactivity

Two forces act within the nucleus, the repulsive electrostatic force between the positively charged protons and the short range attractive nuclear force between protons and neutrons. Sometimes conflicting forces cause the atom to become unstable and this results in the emission of radiation.

The term *radiation* is used to describe a variety of emissions, some of which are electromagnetic waves while others are streams of particles (*see* Chapter 3). These radiations were first discovered by the French physicist Becquerel in 1896. He found that photographic plates stored in a closed drawer had become fogged. Also in the drawer were some crystals of uranium and the shadows on the plates corresponded to the shape of the uranium crystals. (This is an example of serendipity, the faculty of making happy discoveries by accident.) There followed intensive research into the nature of this radiation and it was a very simple experiment which provided the answer.

The Nature of Radioactivity

A narrow beam of emission from uranium was allowed to pass through a magnetic field. This revealed three different types of radiation, one positively charged, one negatively charged and one neutral (*see* Fig. 4.5). Following subsequent experiments the emissions were classified as alpha particles, beta particles and gamma rays, all examples of 'ionizing radiations' (*see* Chapter 3).

Rutherford and others, from their experiments, believed radioactivity to be the result of the spontaneous decay or disintegration of an atom, causing the atom to shoot out an alpha or beta particle with the release of surplus energy in the form of kinetic energy (*see* Chapter 2) and gamma rays.

Alpha Particles

Alpha particles are helium atoms which have lost both their electrons to form helium ions (that is ions with a double-positive electric charge having lost two electrons). The remaining protons and neutrons are strongly bound together in the helium nucleus.

Beta Particles

Beta particles are electrons which may be travelling at a rate approaching the speed of light $(3 \times 10^8 \text{ m s}^{-1})$. These electrons arise when an unstable neutron breaks down into a proton and an electron. When a neutron undergoes this transformation the electron is promptly emitted from the nucleus as a beta particle and the proton is retained.

Gamma Rays

Gamma radiation is a form of electromagnetic radiation of very short wavelength, shorter even than that of X-rays.

Other Emissions

Other emissions can occur in the process of radioactive decay, although less frequently. These include neutrons, protons, deutrons, positrons and nutrinos (*see* Glossary).

Work by the Curies and others showed uranium to be only one of a number of naturally occurring radioactive elements. We

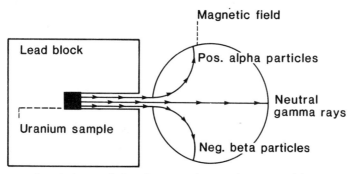

Fig. 4.5 Types of emission radiating from uranium and separated in a magnetic field.

now know that radioactive isotopes of stable atoms also exist, for example carbon-14, which is present in the cells of all living things.

Transmutations other than naturally occurring ones can be brought into being by bombardment of nuclei with sub-atomic particles. It is by this method that nuclides of new elements which do not occur naturally are created. The elements neptunium and plutonium were the first such man-made elements.

Similar reactions have produced radioactive isotopes of nuclides of elements that occur naturally as stable atoms. These isotopes can be mixed with naturally occurring samples of the same element and used as *tracers* for chemical and biological research and medical research and investigation.

Laws of Radioactive Decay
When a nuclide decays and emits an alpha particle its atomic number is decreased by 2 and its mass number by 4. Beta emission causes the atomic number to increase by 1 but the mass number is unchanged.

A nuclide must therefore change into another nuclide following the emission of a particle. For example, uranium, atomic number 92, contains 92 protons and 146 neutrons. After emission of an alpha particle it will contain 90 protons and 144 neutrons. 90 is the atomic number of the element thorium. Radioactive carbon, atomic number 6, contains 6 protons and 14 neutrons. After emission of a beta particle it will contain 7 protons and 14 neutrons. 7 is the atomic number of the element nitrogen.

Atoms of all elements which have an atomic number greater than 82 (lead) are found to be unstable. This has led to the suggestion that the maximum possible size of atomic nuclei is limited. All nuclides with an atomic number greater than 82 are radioactive. Products of radioactive emissions may themselves be radioactive. From one parent nuclide a number of emissions may be required before a stable nucleus is produced.

It is not yet known what causes a particular atom to disintegrate at a particular time. It is known to be entirely random. Decay is not influenced by the physical state of a substance, that is whether it exists as a solid, liquid or gas, and it occurs whether the element is in its pure state or in chemical combination with another element. Nothing can start or stop the process and its speed cannot be increased or retarded. Every radioactive substance has a definite rate of decay. This rate, which depends on the number of atoms present in the sample, is known as the *half-life*.

Half-life
The half-life (symbol $t_{1/2}$) period of a radioactive substance is defined as the time taken for half of the atoms present in the sample to decay. This can vary from 10^{-12} s to 10^{10} years. Radium has a half-life of 1620 years: i.e. in a sample containing 1 g of radium, 0.5 g will have decayed in 1620 years. Uranium-238, the naturally occurring parent of a whole series of emissions leading to the stable element lead, has a half-life of 4.5×10^9 years. Radioactive iodine has a half-life of only 8 days.

Chemical Properties of Elements
It is in the nature of science to observe, measure, classify, correlate and predict. It is not surprising, therefore, that scientists have looked for, and found, relationships between elements. The periodic table of the elements (*see* Fig. 4.6), originally formulated by Mendeleev, indicates that elements of various families or groups possess similar properties. Study of the electronic structure of atoms reveals a rational explanation for these relationships, as well as showing how electronic interactions allow atoms to combine. Theories of chemical bonding and electronic structure enable predictions about the properties of chemicals to be made (*see* Chapter 5).

Periodicity
Elements set out in horizontal rows in order of their atomic number can be arranged in a pattern or table that brings together elements with similar chemical properties. This pattern is known as the 'Periodic Table' (*Figure* 4.6) because elements with similar properties appear at regular and predictable intervals. This periodic relationship was first discovered by Dmitri Mendeleev (1834–1907). Although unaware of the existence of protons and neutrons, Mendeleev *was* aware that the atoms

Groups → 1A

Transition Elements

Period	1A	2A	3B	4B	5B	6B	7B	8B	8B	8B	1B	2B	3A	4A	5A	6A	7A	0
1	1 H																	2 He
2	3 Li	4 Be											5 B	6 C	7 N	8 O	9 F	10 Ne
3	11 Na	12 Mg											13 Al	14 Si	15 P	16 S	17 Cl	18 Ar
4	19 K	20 Ca	21 Sc	22 Ti	23 V	24 Cr	25 Mn	26 Fe	27 Co	28 Ni	29 Cu	30 Zn	31 Ga	32 Ge	33 As	34 Se	35 Br	36 Kr
5	37 Rb	38 Sr	39 Y	40 Zr	41 Nb	42 Mo	43 Tc	44 Ru	45 Rh	46 Pd	47 Ag	48 Cd	49 In	50 Sn	51 Sb	52 Te	53 I	54 Xe
6	55 Cs	56 Ba	57 to 71	72 Hf	73 Ta	74 W	75 Re	76 Os	77 Ir	78 Pt	79 Au	80 Hg	81 Ti	82 Pb	83 Bi	84 Po	85 At	86 Ra
7	87 Fr	88 Ra	89 to 103	104 Rf	105 Ha	106												

Periods ↑

Lanthanide Series

57 La	58 Ce	59 Pr	60 Nd	61 Pm	62 Sm	63 Eu	64 Gd	65 Tb	66 Dy	67 Ho	68 Er	69 Tm	70 Yb	71 Lu

Actinide Series

89 Ac	90 Th	91 Pa	92 U	93 Np	94 Pu	95 Am	96 Cm	97 Bk	98 Cf	99 Es	100 Fm	101 Md	102 No	103 Lw

Fig. 4.6 The Periodic Table. Each square represents an element which is denoted by its atomic number and chemical symbol.

of each element differ in atomic weight and that atomic weight increased at a regular and progressive rate. He wrote the names and weights of all known elements on to cards and spent two years shuffling the cards around and eventually found the pattern in which elements in vertical columns had similar chemical properties. This was the first periodic table. By using blank cards he was able to predict the weight and chemical properties of elements yet to be discovered.

Properties

When Mendeleev spoke of similar 'properties' he was referring to such things as the formation of oxides (compounds with oxygen), hydrides (compounds with hydrogen) and chlorides (compounds with chlorine). In the formation of such compounds elements of different groups adhere to the same general formula. For instance, two atoms of a Group I element will combine with one atom of oxygen to form an oxide (R_2O). One atom of a Group I element will combine with one atom of chlorine to form a chloride (RCl). *Table* 4.4 shows how the elements of each different group adhere to the same general formula.

Table 4.4 General formulae of compounds

Group	Compound	General formula
I	Oxides	R_2O
I	Chlorides	RCl
II	Oxides	RO
II	Chlorides	RCl_2
IV	Oxides	RO_2
IV	Chlorides	RCl_4

It has since been shown that periodicity, the periodic law, reflects the arrangement of electrons in the outer shells of atoms and that elements with the same number of electrons in their outermost shell have similar chemical properties (*see* Chapter 5). The discovery of the interior structure of the atom in the 1930s proved the accuracy of Mendeleev's table. Moreover by this time the elements whose existence he had predicted had been discovered.

Since 1934 scientists have created elements by bombarding an element with neutrons and so transforming it into an element of the next higher atomic number. These are called the *transuranic elements* and so far 14 such elements have been created.

There are eight main groups of typical elements. Some are known by their common name, such as Group I the alkali metals, Group II the alkali earth metals, Group VII the halogens, Group 0 the Noble gases.

The Modern Periodic Table

The modern Periodic Table is organized into horizontal *Periods* and vertical *Groups* which show a marked similarity to each other and form distinct chemical families. Group 1A, the alkali metals, are all soft metals which decompose water and liberate oxygen and form alkaline solutions. Moving from left to right, the elements become less metallic in nature and eventually become non-metals such as carbon, sulphur and chlorine. The Group 0 elements are all unreactive inert gases.

The transition elements in the B group show a relatively gradual change in properties. Their similarity can be explained in terms of their electron structure, as when they take part in chemical reactions (Chapter 5) it is the penultimate electron shell rather than the usual outer electron shell which is filling up. They are all heavy metals with high melting and boiling points, they readily form alloys with one another and are excellent catalysts.

The lanthanides (rare earths) and actinides do not conform to the general pattern and can be considered as a transition series within a transition series. They are all metals and their compounds are often strongly coloured. They can form more than one compound with other elements. For example, chlorine can combine with copper as $CuCl_2$ and as $CuCl$, it can also combine with iron as $FeCl_3$, which is yellow brown in colour, and as $FeCl_2$ which is green. The lanthanides, atomic numbers 57–71, have properties which resemble those of aluminium. The actinides, atomic number 89–103, are noted for their radioactivity; they include the three naturally occurring elements thorium, protactinium and uranium and 11 artificial, or man-made elements.

5

Electrons and chemical bonds

The way in which orbiting electrons are arranged in spherical layers or shells has been mentioned in Chapter 4. Electrons will remain at a predictable distance from the nucleus but they tend to fly about in all directions, creating a three-dimensional 'cloud' of electrical charge (the 'cloud of probability').

Each shell can only hold a certain number of electrons; for instance the first, innermost, shell can hold only 2, the second, 8 and the third, 18. The outermost shell can never hold more than 8 electrons and the greatest possible number of shells an atom can have is 7. Shells are identified by the letters K to Q, K being the innermost shell.

Electronic Configurations

The electronic configuration of an atom can be expressed by stating the number of electrons in each succeeding shell (see Table 5.1). Hydrogen, which has a single electron, is expressed as K1 or simply as 1. Lithium, which has 3 electrons, 2 in the innermost shell and one in the second, is expressed as K2.L1, or simply 2.1. Neon, with its 10 electrons, has 2 in the first shell and 8 in the second, so is expressed 2.8. Elements with more than 10 electrons will use additional shells. Sodium, for instance, has 11 electrons and is expressed as 2.8.1., and argon, with 18 electrons, as 2.8.8.

Potassium has 19 electrons, so the electronic configuration might be expected to be 2.8.9., but because the outermost shell cannot hold more than 8 electrons, a fourth shell will be started and the configuration will be 2.8.8.1.

The outermost shell of all elements in a particular group will contain the same number of electrons. For instance, all Group I elements will have only one electron in their outermost shell, so potassium, the example given above, conforms to the configuration of elements in Group I.

Each shell is differentiated into various energy levels (see p.34). Each energy level in turn contains a certain number of *orbitals* which can hold a maximum of two electrons. These orbitals are divided into four types, s,p,d,f, each of which has its own characteristic shape and can hold a maximum number of paired electrons (see Table 5.2).

Electron Spin

Within their shells electrons spin, but only in two directions. These can be thought of as being clockwise and anti-clockwise. Electrons with opposite spins form stable pairs and this property of pairing is important in chemical reactions.

Successive Ionizing Energies

Electrons in the outermost shell have the highest energy level and are the most easily removed. It is these electrons which are involved in chemical reactions.

Energy (see Chapter 2) is needed to remove an electron and each time this happens relatively more energy will be required to remove the next one. When one electron is removed from, say, a sodium atom (atomic number 11), only 10 electrons (hence 10 negative electrical charges) remain, but there will still be 11 protons with positive charges. In such a positively charged ion (cation) the greater positive charge of the nucleus will bind

Table 5.1 The arrangement of electrons in atoms

Atomic number	Element	K 1s	L 2s	L 2p	M 3s	M 3p	M 3d	N 4s	N 4p	N 4d	N 4f	O 5s
1	H	1										
2	He	2										
3	Li	2	1									
4	Be	2	2									
5	B	2	2	1								
6	C	2	2	2								
7	N	2	2	3								
8	O	2	2	4								
9	F	2	2	5								
10	Ne	2	2	6								
11	Na	2	2	6	1							
12	Mg	2	2	6	2							
13	Al	2	2	6	2	1						
14	Si	2	2	6	2	2						
15	P	2	2	6	2	3						
16	S	2	2	6	2	4						
17	Cl	2	2	6	2	5						
18	Ar	2	2	6	2	6						
19	K	2	2	6	2	6		1				
20	Ca	2	2	6	2	6		2				
21	Sc	2	2	6	2	6	1	2				
22	Ti	2	2	6	2	6	2	2				
23	V	2	2	6	2	6	3	2				
24	Cr	2	2	6	2	6	5	1				
25	Mn	2	2	6	2	6	5	2				
26	Fe	2	2	6	2	6	6	2				
27	Co	2	2	6	2	6	7	2				
28	Ni	2	2	6	2	6	8	2				
29	Cu	2	2	6	2	6	10	1				
30	Zn	2	2	6	2	6	10	2				
31	Ga	2	2	6	2	6	10	2	1			
32	Ge	2	2	6	2	6	10	2	2			
33	As	2	2	6	2	6	10	2	3			
34	Se	2	2	6	2	6	10	2	4			
35	Br	2	2	6	2	6	10	2	5			
36	Kr	2	2	6	2	6	10	2	6			
37	Rb	2	2	6	2	6	10	2	6			1
38	Sr	2	2	6	2	6	10	2	6			2
39	Y	2	2	6	2	6	10	2	6	1		2
40	Zr	2	2	6	2	6	10	2	6	2		2
41	Nb	2	2	6	2	6	10	2	6	4		1
42	Mo	2	2	6	2	6	10	2	6	5		1
43	Tc	2	2	6	2	6	10	2	6	6		1
44	Ru	2	2	6	2	6	10	2	6	7		1
45	Rh	2	2	6	2	6	10	2	6	8		1
46	Pd	2	2	6	2	6	10	2	6	10		

Table 5.1 (*cont*)

Atomic number	Element	K	L		M			N				O					P				Q	
		1s	2s	2p	3s	3p	3d	4s	4p	4d	4f	5s	5p	5d	5f	5g	6s	6p	6d	6f	7s	7p
47	Ag	2	2	6	2	6	10	2	6	10		1										
48	Cd	2	2	6	2	6	10	2	6	10		2										
49	In	2	2	6	2	6	10	2	6	10		2	1									
50	Sn	2	2	6	2	6	10	2	6	10		2	2									
51	Sb	2	2	6	2	6	10	2	6	10		2	3									
52	Te	2	2	6	2	6	10	2	6	10		2	4									
53	I	2	2	6	2	6	10	2	6	10		2	5									
54	Xe	2	2	6	2	6	10	2	6	10		2	6									
55	Cs	2	2	6	2	6	10	2	6	10		2	6				1					
56	Ba	2	2	6	2	6	10	2	6	10		2	6				2					
57	La	2	2	6	2	6	10	2	6	10		2	6	1			2					
58	Ce	2	2	6	2	6	10	2	6	10	2	2	6				2					
59	Pr	2	2	6	2	6	10	2	6	10	3	2	6				2					
60	Nd	2	2	6	2	6	10	2	6	10	4	2	6				2					
61	Pm	2	2	6	2	6	10	2	6	10	5	2	6				2					
62	Sm	2	2	6	2	6	10	2	6	10	6	2	6				2					
63	Eu	2	2	6	2	6	10	2	6	10	7	2	6				2					
64	Gd	2	2	6	2	6	10	2	6	10	7	2	6	1			2					
65	Tb	2	2	6	2	6	10	2	6	10	9	2	6				2					
66	Dy	2	2	6	2	6	10	2	6	10	10	2	6				2					
67	Ho	2	2	6	2	6	10	2	6	10	11	2	6				2					
68	Er	2	2	6	2	6	10	2	6	10	12	2	6				2					
69	Tm	2	2	6	2	6	10	2	6	10	13	2	6				2					
70	Yb	2	2	6	2	6	10	2	6	10	14	2	6				2					
71	Lu	2	2	6	2	6	10	2	6	10	14	2	6	1			2					
72	Hf	2	2	6	2	6	10	2	6	10	14	2	6	2			2					
73	Ta	2	2	6	2	6	10	2	6	10	14	2	6	3			2					
74	W	2	2	6	2	6	10	2	6	10	14	2	6	4			2					
75	Re	2	2	6	2	6	10	2	6	10	14	2	6	5			2					
76	Os	2	2	6	2	6	10	2	6	10	14	2	6	6			2					
77	Ir	2	2	6	2	6	10	2	6	10	14	2	6	9								
78	Pt	2	2	6	2	6	10	2	6	10	14	2	6	9			1					
79	Au	2	2	6	2	6	10	2	6	10	14	2	6	10			1					
80	Hg	2	2	6	2	6	10	2	6	10	14	2	6	10			2					
81	Ti	2	2	6	2	6	10	2	6	10	14	2	6	10			2	1				
82	Pb	2	2	6	2	6	10	2	6	10	14	2	6	10			2	2				
83	Bi	2	2	6	2	6	10	2	6	10	14	2	6	10			2	3				
84	Po	2	2	6	2	6	10	2	6	10	14	2	6	10			2	4				
85	At	2	2	6	2	6	10	2	6	10	14	2	6	10			2	5				
86	Rn	2	2	6	2	6	10	2	6	10	14	2	6	10			2	6				
87	Fr	2	2	6	2	6	10	2	6	10	14	2	6	10			2	6			1	
88	Ra	2	2	6	2	6	10	2	6	10	14	2	6	10			2	6			2	
89	Ac	2	2	6	2	6	10	2	6	10	14	2	6	10			2	6	1		2	
90	Th	2	2	6	2	6	10	2	6	10	14	2	6	10			2	6	2		2	
91	Pa	2	2	6	2	6	10	2	6	10	14	2	6	10	2		2	6	1		2	
92	U	2	2	6	2	6	10	2	6	10	14	2	6	10	3		2	6	1		2	

The table gives the numbers of electrons in the various shells of the atoms. It refers to neutral atoms in their lowest energy states.

Table 5.2 Types of orbital showing maximum number of paired electrons

Type	Maximum possible orbitals	Equivalent electrons
s	1	2
p	3	6
d	5	10
f	7	14

the remaining electrons more closely, hence the need for relatively more energy to remove each successive electron. These are called *successive ionizing energies*. The first ionizing energy is that required to remove the first electron, the second ionizing energy that required to remove the second, and so on.

The first electron can thus be removed far more easily, that is with less energy, than any of the others. A graph showing the amount of extra energy required to remove each successive electron shows that the electrons fall into three distinct energy groups or 'levels' (*Fig.* 5.1). These energy levels correspond to the shells in which electrons are arranged.

The Danish physicist Niels Bohr was first to point out, in 1913, that atoms can exist in a series of states and that each state has a certain energy level. Generally the atom is most stable when it has minimum energy—when it is in its *ground state*. If the atom absorbs energy in excess of its ground state it is said to be in an *excited state*. Atoms cannot exist between states but they can absorb enough energy to enable them to jump to a higher energy level. When an atom moves from a higher to a lower energy level its surplus

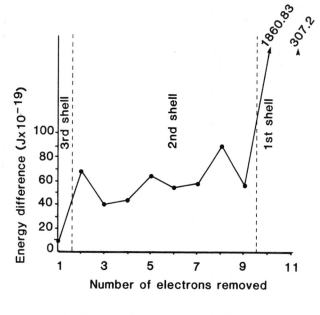

Sodium electron energy shells

Shell 3 •

Shell 2 • • • • • • •

Shell 1 • •

Fig. 5.1 The amount of extra energy required to remove successive electrons from a sodium atom, showqing different energy levels.

energy will be emitted in the form of radiation. If this radiation is in the form of visible light then the atoms from a particular element will all be of the same wavelength and hence of the same colour (*see* Chapter 3). This emission of radiation by excited atoms can occur spontaneously but it can also be induced by other radiations, when all of the atoms present will emit their excess energy very rapidly at the same time. This process is called *Light Amplification by Stimulated Emission of Radiation* or *laser* action.

Unlike ordinary visible light, which spreads out from its source, laser light travels in a perfectly straight line. Even after travelling a distance of 250 000 miles from earth to the moon a laser beam will only have spread a few miles. Laser light is intense because all the waves are in phase (*see* Chapter 3) and so the intensity of the light will be equal to the sum of all the individual intensities.

The ruby laser is the most powerful member of the laser family. It produces a pure red light which is ten million times more powerful than sunlight. Because of the intense heat produced and the precise direction of the beam it can be used in the treatment of skin cancer and of eye conditions such as detached retina and glaucoma.

In surgery, using laser scalpels the size of incisions can be minimized and blood vessels can be cauterized, so reducing blood loss. This is particularly valuable for haemophiliacs. In industry the heat of the laser beam can be used for precision cutting, burning and welding. In civil engineering the perfectly straight laser beam can be used in the construction of tunnels. Lasers are also used in the telecommunications industry (fibre optics) and to create the three dimensional images called holograms.

Simple Theories of Bonding

As we have seen the atom consists of a nucleus surrounded by a cloud of orbiting electrons which are arranged in layers or shells. Each electron shell can only hold a certain maximum number of electrons (first 2, second 8, third 18) and the outermost shell can never hold more than 8. The elements in Group 0 of the

Periodic Table all have the maximum possible number of electrons in their outermost shell. These elements, the Noble gases, are extraordinarily unreactive (inert) because their filled outermost shell makes their electronic structure more stable than that of other elements.

Simple theories of chemical bonding are based on the assumption that elements which do not possess such stable electronic structures seek to attain them by reacting with other elements. Atoms can combine in two main ways, by electron transfer, *ionic* or *electrovalent bonding*, and by electron sharing, *covalent bonding*.

Electrovalent Compounds

Electrons are most easily removed from Group I elements and most difficult to remove from Group VII. Group I elements, the alkali metals, have the electronic structure of a Noble gas plus one electron (*see Table* 5.1). They can therefore attain the electronic configuration (structure) of a Noble gas by the loss of one electron. For example, the loss of one electron from the lithium atom (2.1.) will produce a positive lithium ion with the electronic structure of the Noble gas helium (2.).

Group V elements, the halogens, have the electronic structure of a Noble gas less one electron. They will attain the electronic configuration of a Noble gas by the addition of one electron. For example, fluorine (2.7.), by gaining an electron, attains the electronic structure of neon (2.8.).

All elements of Groups I, II and III form positive ions which retain the name of the element (lithium, beryllium, boron etc). Elements of Groups VI and VII form negative ions and the name of the element changes to end in 'ide' (oxide, sulphide, fluoride, chloride etc.). Ions of opposite charge will be attracted and will form electrovalent bonds. For example, positive ions of lithium will combine with negative ions of chloride to form lithium chloride (*see Fig.* 5.2).

Elements of Groups IV and V do not normally form ions because too much energy is needed for the atoms to gain or lose so many electrons.

The ion does not retain the properties of the parent atom. Sodium, for instance, is a soft silvery metal which burns freely in air and reacts vigorously with water. Chlorine is a greenish yellow poisonous gas with a pungent smell. In combination the sodium and chloride ions form sodium chloride, which is familiar to us all as common salt. It is important to remember this when considering the toxic effects of various substances because chemicals used as raw materials may well change their properties and become more or less toxic when they react with other chemicals. The same applies to chemicals taken into the human body, itself a chemical processing plant, as these can react with the chemicals which are already present. Electrovalent compounds are also known as 'ionic compounds' for the obvious reason that they are a combination of ions.

Covalent Compounds
Many molecules are formed by the sharing rather than the transfer of electrons, one electron from each atom making up the pair which forms a *covalent bond*. In this way elements which do not normally form ions can combine. For example, carbon (2.4) would need to shed 4 electrons to attain the electronic configuration of helium (2) and in terms of energy expenditure this would be grossly un-economic. However, by gaining 4 electrons

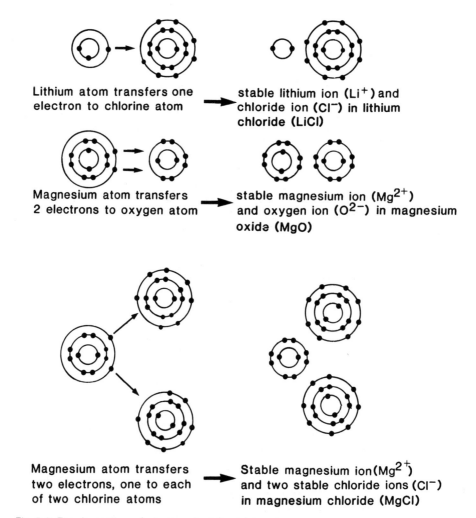

Lithium atom transfers one electron to chlorine atom → stable lithium ion (Li^+) and chloride ion (Cl^-) in lithium chloride (LiCl)

Magnesium atom transfers 2 electrons to oxygen atom → stable magnesium ion (Mg^{2+}) and oxygen ion (O^{2-}) in magnesium oxide (MgO)

Magnesium atom transfers two electrons, one to each of two chlorine atoms → Stable magnesium ion (Mg^{2+}) and two stable chloride ions (Cl^-) in magnesium chloride (MgCl)

Fig. 5.2 The formation of electrovalent (ionic) bonds.

carbon can attain the electronic configuration of neon (2.8) and it does this by sharing 4 electrons with other atoms.

Carbon tetrachloride is one of the many known carbon compounds and each molecule is composed of one carbon atom and 4 (tetra) chlorine atoms. Covalent bonds can also be formed by atoms which *do* normally form ions. Fluorine (2.7) for example needs to gain one electron to attain the electronic configuration of neon (2.8). It can do this by sharing one of its electrons with an electron from another fluorine atom to form a molecule of fluorine (*see Fig.* 5.3).

Covalent bonds also produce macro-molecules (Chapter 11), the giant molecules wherein the structure continues indefinitely.

Co-ordinate Bonding

This is a type of covalent bonding where the pair of shared electrons are both donated by the same atom, the other atom supplying none. This type of bonding is found in boron tri-fluoride (BF_3) and in ammonia (NH_3).

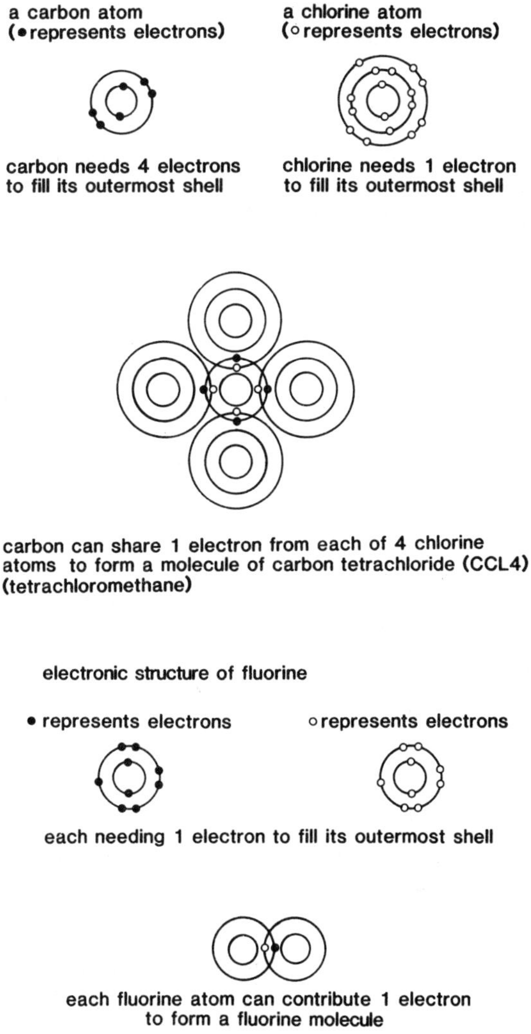

a carbon atom
(• represents electrons)

a chlorine atom
(○ represents electrons)

carbon needs 4 electrons
to fill its outermost shell

chlorine needs 1 electron
to fill its outermost shell

carbon can share 1 electron from each of 4 chlorine
atoms to form a molecule of carbon tetrachloride (CCL4)
(tetrachloromethane)

electronic structure of fluorine

• represents electrons   ○ represents electrons

each needing 1 electron to fill its outermost shell

each fluorine atom can contribute 1 electron
to form a fluorine molecule

Fig. 5.3 The formation of covalent compounds.

Characteristics of Electrovalent Compounds

In these compounds atoms will be arranged in a three-dimensional lattice in which strong electrostatic forces hold the atoms together. In order to break these bonds a great deal of energy is required, which explains why these compounds generally have high melting and boiling points. They do not conduct electricity in their solid state but they do when they are dissolved or dissociated into ions in solution. They are often soluble in water but virtually all are insoluble in non-polar liquids such as petrol, benzene, carbon tetrachloride. (In non-polar liquids bonds are covalent rather than ionic.) As a general rule, polar liquids dissolve ionic compounds whilst non-polar liquids dissolve covalent compounds—'like dissolves like'. Sodium chloride is an ionic compound which exhibits these properties. It does not melt easily and does not conduct electricity in its solid state, but a solution wherein sodium and chloride ions have dissociated is a good conductor of electricity (Chapter 6). It is soluble in water but not in petrol, benzene or carbon tetrachloride.

These characteristic properties occur because in electrovalent (ionic) compounds there are no discrete molecules as there are in covalent compounds. Sodium chloride for instance is merely an assembly of positive and negative ions with a ratio of sodium to chloride of $1:1$.

Characteristics of Covalent Compounds

Most covalent compounds are composed of discrete molecules in which the atoms are bound together by powerful forces but the forces between the molecules are weak. For instance, crystalline iodine is shown by X-ray diffraction to consist of pairs of atoms separated by relatively short distances. Because of the weak bonds between the molecules they have low melting and boiling points. At room pressure and temperature they are likely to be gases, volatile liquids or low melting points solids. Not all covalent compounds are volatile however, nor do they all consist of discrete molecules. Diamond and quartz are such exceptions.

Solubility in water is low, although some are hydrolysed in water. They usually dissolve in non-polar or organic liquids (petrol, benzene, carbon tetrachloride).

Valency

The number of bonds that a particular atom can make is known as its *valency* and the electron which takes part in a chemical reaction is known as the valency electron.

Monovalent atoms, such as sodium and chlorine, have a valency of 1. They form compounds of the type $NaCl$; compounds of the type Na_2Cl or $NaCl_2$ cannot exist.

Divalent atoms, such as magnesium, calcium, oxygen, have a valency of 2. With sodium or chlorine they form compounds such as NaO_2 or $MgCl_2$. They can also combine with each other to form compounds such as MgO. Compounds such as $MgCl$ or Mg_2O cannot exist.

Trivalent compounds, such as aluminium and boron, have a valency of 3. With hydroxyl molecules aluminium will form compounds of the type $Al(OH_3)$. Boron with fluoride will form boron trifluoride, BF_3.

Electrovalency

Electrovalency is the term used to indicate the number of electrons an atom needs to shed or acquire in order to attain the electronic configuration of a Noble gas (*see Table* 5.3).

Table 5.3 Electrovalency of atoms in various groups

Group	Electrons to add	Electrons to lose	Electro-valency
I	1		1
II	2		2
III	3		3
VII		1	−1
VI		2	−2

Covalency States

Covalency state is the term used to indicate the number of paired electrons needed to form a molecule (*see Table* 5.4).

Electron sharing and electron transfer have been presented as separated entities but this is a simplification. The two types of bonding would be better considered as extremes, the true formation being somewhere between the two.

Table 5.4 Covalency states of some molecules

Molecule	Shared electrons	Covalency state
Fluoride gas (F_2)	2 (1 pair)	1
Water (H_2O)	4 (2 pairs)	2
Ammonia (NH_3)	6 (3 pairs)	3
Methane (CH_4)	8 (4 pairs)	4

Hydrogen Bonds

In some covalent compounds such as water (H_2O) the shared electron clouds tend to be more concentrated at one end of the molecule than the other. For example, in the water molecule the result is a small negative charge at the oxygen end and a small positive charge at the hydrogen end. This is known as 'polarity' and it causes an additional weak electrostatic bond *between* molecules. It is an effect that occurs only with molecules containing hydrogen (in combination with oxygen, fluorine, nitrogen or chlorine) and hence it is called a *hydrogen bond*.

These bonds, which are encountered between (intermolecular) rather than within molecules (intramolecular), cause the compounds in which they are found to have a higher melting and boiling point than would be expected. For instance, without hydrogen bonding water would be a gas at room temperature. Hydrogen bonding also accounts for the formation of hydrates, compounds which contain molecules of water, such as cupric sulphate (copper sulphate) ($CuSO_4$).

Bonds in Metals and Metallic Compounds

All metals share similar characteristics. They are all opaque and have a metallic lustre. They are malleable, i.e. they can be hammered into shape, and ductile, can be drawn into wires. They are good conductors of heat and electricity.

The position of the metals in the Periodic Table is significant. The fact that they are all concentrated in one broad area suggests that their metallic characteristics may be related to electronic structure. Metals are thought to contain electrons which move freely through the body of the metal. These are known as 'free electrons' (*see Fig.* 5.4).

Ductility and malleability are explained by the fact that the ions, being of a like charge, are able to slip over each other in several directions. Metallic lustre, which is associated with mobile electrons, is lost when metals are vaporized. Vapours of mercury, zinc and sodium do not conduct electricity; they are monatomic (consisting of one atom only) and metallic bonds are absent.

Molecular Shapes

Atoms are not free to position themselves in a molecule in any random manner. Electrons carry a negative electrical charge, and like charges repel (*see* Chapter 6). According to the electron pair repulsion theory, it is because of this that the electron pairs in the valency shells of atoms try to get as far apart as possible. Consequently the shapes of molecules vary according to the number of negative charges 'repelling' each other.

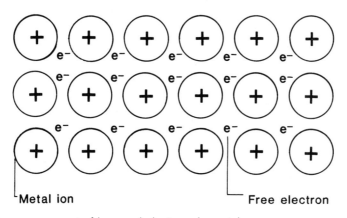

Fig. 5.4 The arrangement of ions and electrons in metal.

Each type of molecule will have its own particular shape, the simplest being the linear and the tetrahedral (*see Fig.* 5.5).

Shapes range from these simple ones to the highly complex double helix of deoxyribonucleic acid (DNA) (*see Fig.* 5.6).

Biological systems depend almost entirely on the existence of these specific and defined shapes. This is particularly true of enzymes, which are the keys to many of the chemical reactions of metabolism. The action of enzymes is very specific and depends on molecular shape—the key must fit.

Compounds and Mixtures

A chemical *compound* is a substance that consists of two or more elements that are chemically united. It contains only molecules of that compound and cannot be broken down into simpler substances without breaking the chemical bond. In other words, it cannot change unless a chemical reaction occurs.

Mixtures differ from compounds because they consist of two or more substances which are not chemically united. They can therefore readily be separated into their components using appropriate physical or mechanical means. For example sea water is a mixture of water and minerals, air is a mixture of gases and blood is a mixture of complex chemical compounds. The formation and separation of mixtures, unlike the formation and separation of chemical compounds, does not involve either the absorption or the production of heat energy.

Chemical Reactions

Symbols are used to simplify the writing of elements and chemical reactions. Those unfamiliar with these symbols may find it useful to refer to Appendix 5 before proceeding with this section.

Characteristics of Chemical Change

Chemical reactions are occurring constantly: for example, when fuel burns, when adhesives set, when food is eaten. The following characteristics are common to all chemical reactions.

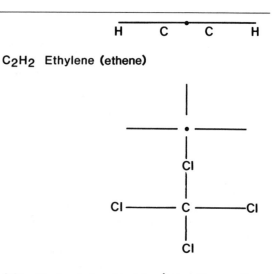

C_2H_2 Ethylene (ethene)

CCl_4 Carbontetrachloride (tetrachloromethane)

Fig. 5.5 Linear and tetrahedral molecules.

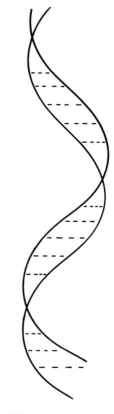

Fig. 5.6 The double helix of DNA.

● Whenever a chemical reaction occurs the original substances (reactants) are changed into different substances (products) and the properties of the products will differ from those of the reactants.

● During any chemical reaction matter can neither be created nor destroyed so the weight (mass) of the products must equal the weight (mass) of the reactants.

● In any chemical reaction energy is either given out or absorbed. For instance, when carbon burns in oxygen, energy is given out in the form of heat and light. However if sulphur is to combine with carbon to form carbon disulphide, then heat must be added. Reactions in which heat is liberated are termed *exothermic*. Reactions which require heat to be added are termed *endothermic*. In a few reactions heat is neither added nor given off and these reactions are called *athermic*.

Some Types of Chemical Reaction
Synthesis
The combination of two or more substances to form a single substance is called *synthesis* or combination. Synthesis has only *one product*. For example:

iron　　+ sulphur → iron sulphide
(Fe　　+　S　→　　FeS)

nitrogen　+ hydrogen →　ammonia
(N_2　　+　$3H_2$　→　　$2NH_3$)

Decomposition
Decomposition is the opposite of synthesis. It occurs when a single substance is broken down into two or more simpler substances. Decomposition has only *one reactant*. For example:

calcium carbonate + heat → calcium oxide
+ carbon dioxide
($CaCO_3$　　+　heat　→　$CaO + CO_2$)

Combustion
Combustion usually means the reaction of a substance with oxygen, when heat and light will be given off. For example:

magnesium　+ oxygen → magnesium oxide
($2Mg$　　+　O_2　→　　$2MgO$)

This reaction gives out heat and white light and so is exothermic. It is used for distress flares and fireworks. The burning of gas, coal, petrol and oil are all examples of combustion, the heat produced being a valuable source of energy.

Precipitation
Some solutions, when mixed together, react to give an insoluble product and this product appears as a *suspension* or *precipitation*. For example, from a solution of sodium chloride (NaCl) mixed with a solution of silver nitrate ($AgNO_3$), silver chloride (AgCl) will be precipitated because it is insoluble. The sodium nitrate, being soluble, will remain in solution. The equation for this reaction would read:

$$AgNO_3 + NaCl → AgCl↓ + NaNO_3$$

Displacement
During some reactions an element from one compound will be displaced by another. For instance, if iron and copper are competing to exist in the same solution iron will 'win' because it is more reactive than copper. If an iron nail is placed in a copper sulphate solution (which is blue) a coat of copper will appear on the nail and the solution will change colour from blue to pale green.

iron　+ copper sulphate → iron sulphate
+ copper
(Fe　+　$CuSO_4$　→ $FeSO_4 + Cu$)

Oxidation and Reduction
Oxidation can be defined as a reaction in which a substance gains oxygen and loses hydrogen. For example, magnesium is oxidized by gaining oxygen:

$$2Mg　+　O_2　→　2MgO$$

Similarly, reduction can be defined as the opposite process, a reaction in which a substance loses oxygen and gains hydrogen. For example nitrogen by gaining hydrogen is reduced to ammonia:

$$N_2　+　3H_2　→　2NH_3$$

Further growth of chemical knowledge has, however, shown these definitions to be somewhat simplistic because oxygen and hydrogen are not always involved in such reactions. It is more useful therefore to define oxidation and reduction in terms of electron loss or gain. If a substance loses electrons during a reaction it has been oxidized, if electrons are gained, then the substance has been reduced.

A closer look at the oxidation of magnesium in terms of electron transfer will show that during the reaction the magnesium atom loses two electrons and the oxygen atom gains two electrons. In other words, magnesium has been oxidized and oxygen reduced.

Oxidation and reduction can occur together and this is known as a *redox reaction*.

Oxidation State

The oxidation state indicates the number of electrons which must be added to a positive ion or removed from a negative ion to get a neutral atom. For example, the iron ion Fe^{2+} needs to gain two electrons to become neutral and so has an oxidation state of 2. The chloride ion Cl^{1-} needs to lose one electron to become neutral and so has an oxidation state of 1.

In covalent molecules it is assumed that the electrons in the bond go to the atom which is most electronegative. In ammonia (NH_3), nitrogen is more electronegative so it is assumed that one electron from each hydrogen atom will go to the nitrogen, which thus had an oxidation state of -3 while hydrogen has an oxidation state of $+1$.

Predicting Reactions

Because any given atom will almost always form a fixed and characteristic number of bonds with other atoms, it is possible to make theoretical predictions about the formulae of compounds. However, the fact that a compound has been shown to be theoretically possible does not mean that that compound does, or can, exist: this can only be proved by experiment. Experiments are expensive, and so the prediction that a particular combination of atoms is *not* possible is valuable in terms of time and money.

Rate of Reactions

Chemical reactions do not all take place at the same rate. Explosions that occur when gas is heated are reactions that are virtually instantaneous. Other reactions, for instance the reaction of iron with oxygen in the presence of water (rusting), is very slow. Rates of reaction can be altered by changing concentrations of reactants, changing pressure and particularly by changing temperature. For example, lowering the temperature of many foodstuffs, by refrigeration, will slow down the rate of decay. The human body, which functions most effectively at 37 °C, will respond to a rise in body temperature by altering the rate of many biochemical reactions—a rise of 6–7 °C is unlikely to be tolerated for long!

In general, increasing the concentration of reactants will increase the rate of reaction. When reactants are gaseous, increasing pressure will result in an increase in the rate of reaction.

Catalysts

A *catalyst* is a substance that will alter the rate of a chemical reaction, although the catalyst itself remains unchanged. Usually only very small quantities of a catalyst are required to initiate or greatly to increase the rate of a reaction. Catalysts are widely used in the chemical industry. Frequently they are metals or oxides of metals. Enzymes are catalysts which are produced by living cells.

Biochemical Reactions

The chemical change which take place in living cells is called metabolism (*see* Chapter 2). Many different changes are taking place at any one time; for instance the production of energy from food, the excretion of waste products, cell growth and cell reproduction. Cellular respiration—the conversion of glucose to energy—itself involves over 70 reactions.

Physical Change

A substance can also undergo physical change, but in this case no new substances are formed. For example, ice, water and steam are all forms of H_2O, the changes being brought about by changes in temperature. Unlike chemical changes, physical changes are usually easily reversed. Chapter 8 considers physical states in more detail.

6

Electricity

A constant and plentiful supply of electricity is something which inhabitants of today's 'high tech' world take very much for granted. The exploitation of electricity is a relatively recent achievement, although man has known of its existence for more than 2000 years. Only from the middle of the nineteenth century have attempts been made to harness its power.

Electricity can now be used in countless ways. It provides light and warmth, power for industrial processes and communication systems to name but a few. Unlike other power sources, such as coal or oil, it can be readily transported from point of source to consumer and is instantly available at the touch of a switch.

Electricity in Nature

In nature it is the power of electricity which holds atomic particles together. Electrical charges are involved in the chemical and physical activity of living organisms, although these charges are not usually detectable without sophisticated apparatus, except in organisms such as the electric eel. The most dramatic form of naturally occurring electrical activity is the flash of lightning.

Static Electricity

When a piece of amber is rubbed with a dry cloth, a force is produced which causes small particles of the cloth to adhere to the amber. The ancient Greeks were undoubtedly amongst the first to create electricity in this way and it was they who named this force *elektron*, the Greek word meaning amber. This word, adapted as *electron*, is used today to describe the sub-atomic particles which are now known to cause this phenomenon.

Electrostatic Force

All matter is composed of atoms, each of which is comprised of an electrically charged nucleus surrounded by electrically charged orbiting electrons (*see* Chapter 4). The positive charge of the nucleus is usually equal in strength to the negative charge of the orbiting electrons, so electrons are normally bound to their parent atom by an *electrostatic force*.

When the piece of amber is rubbed with a cloth this force is overcome because the heat generated by friction is sufficient to allow the outermost electrons to break free from the cloth. They then become attached to the amber, creating a build up of static electric charge. This in turn will attract any other 'spare' electrons such as those of small specks of dust, rather like a magnet picking up iron filings.

The removal of electrons by friction forms the basis of all static electricity. The phenomenon occurs when materials such as glass or plastic are polished with a dry cloth. Small particles of fluff will adhere to the surface being polished. It is for this reason that many household polishes now incorporate anti-static agents.

Attraction and Repulsion

Materials such as amber, glass and plastic which can hold a charge do not all build up the same type of charge. Plastic, for example, will become negatively charged, whilst glass becomes positively charged.

43

Attempts to bring similarly charged objects together, two charged plastic rods for instance or two charged glass rods, will fail because like charges repel. However, when two objects of opposite charge are brought together attraction will occur because opposite charges attract. This is the first 'law of electrostatics', that like charges repel, unlike charges attract.

Insulators and Conductors
Substances which become charged when polished include precious stones, crystals, resin and sulphur as well as those already mentioned. Materials such as these which have the ability to hold an electrical charge are called *insulators*.

Those substances which cannot hold a charge are called *conductors*. Metals are good conductors because their electrons are able to move freely through the lattice of atoms (see Chapter 5).

Electric Fields
It is not necessary for two charged objects to be touching for attraction or repulsion to occur. This is because an electrical force exerted by a charged object will extend beyond the confines of that object. Any electric charge will set up an *electric field* in the space surrounding it and a force will be exerted on any charged object which is placed within this field.

The direction of the electric field at any given point is defined as the direction of the force it produces on a positively charged object. Charged objects are called *electrodes*, and an electric field will always exist between two electrodes. The shape and direction of this field will depend on the type of charge, positive or negative, and on the shape of the electrode, for instance a straight or a point electrode. For instance, between two parallel electrodes with unlike charges the shape of the force will be a straight line and the direction will be from the positive to the negative electrode. Between two point electrodes with unlike charges the force assumes a curved shape. Between two point electrodes with like charges (which repel) the force will be deflected away from the electrodes. *Fig.* 6.1 shows how the shapes of electric fields can differ.

Movement of Electrical Charges
Because static electricity stays in one place it is of little practical importance. Electricity only becomes a power to be exploited when there is movement of the charge.

Atmospheric Electricity
Lightning is an electrical discharge between two charged clouds or between a charged cloud and the earth. This, of course, is a very destructive form of electricity, but it is possible to protect buildings from lightning damage by fixing a lightning conductor, a long pointed iron rod, to the highest point of the side of a building, the lower end being buried in the earth. Negative ions are attracted to the iron point and give up their electrons to be discharged, through the rod, to earth. Any positive ions will be repelled upwards and will spread a space charge which will have only a negligible effect in neutralizing any negative charge.

Electrical Potential
The movement of electrons which takes place in a lightning conductor occurs because of a difference of *potential* (electrical pressure) between the conductor and the earth. Just as temperature differences determine the direction of heat flow, and pressure differences the direction of water flow, so electrical potential differences govern the direction of flow of electricity from one point to another. In the living body a potential electrical difference exists between the two sides of a cell membrane. This serves to control the transmission of nerve impulses and the transmission of substances across the cell membrane.

Electric Current
The potential difference between two charged bodies constitutes the energy available to do work (*see* Chapter 2). If the two charges of an electrical potential difference are free to move, they will do so and create an electric current. In other words, for an electric current to flow between two points a potential difference must exist. It is only when electricity can flow in the form of an electric current that electricity becomes a useful power source.

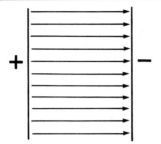 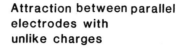

Attraction between parallel
electrodes with
unlike charges

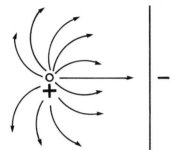

Attraction between straight
and point electrodes with
unlike charges

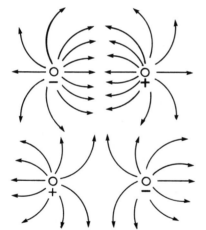

Attraction between point
electrodes with unlike
charges

Repulsion between electrodes
with like charges

Fig. 6.1 The shapes of electrical fields. Arrows indicate the direction of flow.

Electrical Resistance

Electrical resistance is a measure of the property of a material to oppose the flow of a current. It depends on the size (length and thickness of a wire for instance) as well as on the nature of the conductor. The best conductors are those which have the lowest resistance—silver, copper, gold and aluminium.

In their solid state pure metals and graphite are good conductors. Silicon (the silicon chip!) which is important in the computer and electronics industries, conducts electricity less easily and so is known as a *semiconductor*.

Alloys of iron, nickel and chromium have high resistance and are therefore bad conductors. Elements of electric fires are made of these materials because their high electrical resistance and high boiling points allow them to become red hot.

Electricity and the Nervous System

Muscles can be made to contract when stimulated with a mild electric shock. In living tissue this stimulus is transmitted through nerves. There are nerves running from the brain or the spinal cord to every voluntary muscle in the body.

The nerve cell, made up of fibres (axon) surrounded by a protective layer of fatty tissue (myelin), resembles the core of an electric cable surrounded by insulating rubber. Messages pass along this, the nerve axon, in the form of an electric current.

Familiar electric currents occur in two forms; the steady supply required to power such things as light bulbs and the short burst which acts as a signal for a door bell. The current flowing in nerve fibres is of the latter kind, supplying signals not power. A wave of electricity passes down the fibre, with the voltage increasing to a peak then falling as it reaches its destination.

Animal generated electricity, like electricity produced by a battery or generator, is carried by a flow of charged particles. However, in living tissue these particles are positively charged ions rather than negatively charged electrons. The flow is possible because of a potential difference between the two sides of the cell membrane. The inside of the cell maintains a potential 65–95 millivolts (mV) negative to the external surface. This voltage is identical in principle to that produced by a chemical or 'wet' battery.

The electrical activity of the brain can be demonstrated on an electroencephalogram (EEG). A wide spectrum of frequences is present and these have been divided into alpha (8–12 s), beta (18+ s), theta (4–7 s) and delta (1–3.5 s). The pattern of waves depends on many factors, such as age and the area of the brain being studied. The EEG is used clinically to investigate pathological cerebral conditions.

The electrocardiogram (ECG) records the electrical activity of the heart. It can be used to study disturbances in the generation and transmission of the cardiac impulse. An electric shock is sometimes administered to restore normal cardiac rhythm. Electrodes from the apparatus, known as the defibrillator, can be placed either on the chest wall or directly on to the heart.

Electroconvulsive therapy (ECT) is a method of treatment in which a series of brief electrical shocks is administered via electrodes placed on the skull. It has in the past been used in the treatment of many mental disorders but current evidence suggests that it is beneficial only to severely depressed patients.

Chemical Energy and Electricity

When a wire is attached to two rods, one of copper and one of zinc, and both rods immersed in a dilute sulphuric acid solution, an electric current will flow along the wire. This happens because when pure sulphuric acid is added to water, the sulphate group of atoms will separate from the hydrogen taking one electron from each hydrogen atom. The hydrogen atoms therefore become positively charged ions and the sulphate group negatively charged ions. This ionization of sulphuric acid in water can be simply represented by the equation:

$$H_2SO_4 \rightarrow 2H^+ + SO_4^{2-}$$

Zinc slowly dissolves in sulphuric acid to form zinc ions which each leave two electrons behind, thus the zinc rod becomes negatively charged. These electrons are the source of the electric current. Zinc ions are attracted into the solution by the sulphate ions. Hydrogen ions are deposited on the copper plate where they receive an electron from the copper and so are liberated in the form of bubbles of hydrogen gas. In losing the electrons to hydrogen, copper becomes positively charged and so attracts electrons from the zinc causing an electric current to flow through the connecting wires. In this way chemical energy is converted to electrical energy (see Fig. 6.2).

The zinc/copper in acid is an example of the many combinations of acid and metal that can be used to produce a battery capable of converting stored chemical energy into electrical energy. The acid does not necessarily have to be in liquid form, it can be in the form of a moist paste which will minimize the risk of spillage. Dry cell batteries used for torches and portable radios contain acid in this form.

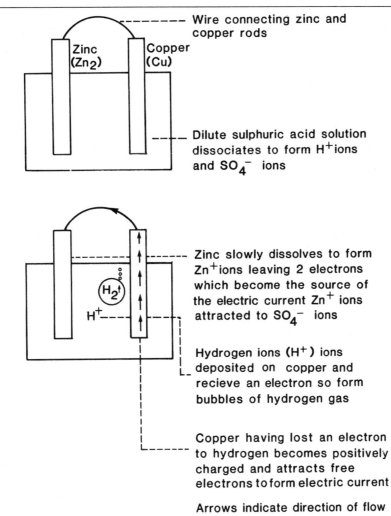

Wire connecting zinc and copper rods

Zinc (Zn_2)

Copper (Cu)

Dilute sulphuric acid solution dissociates to form H^+ ions and SO_4^- ions

Zinc slowly dissolves to form Zn^+ ions leaving 2 electrons which become the source of the electric current Zn^+ ions attracted to SO_4^- ions

Hydrogen ions (H^+) ions deposited on copper and recieve an electron so form bubbles of hydrogen gas

Copper having lost an electron to hydrogen becomes positively charged and attracts free electrons to form electric current

Arrows indicate direction of flow

Fig. 6.2 Conversion of chemical to electrical energy. Arrows indicate direction of electron flow.

Electrolysis

Metals conduct electricity because their electrons are free to move through the lattice of atoms. Molten metals conduct for the same reason. Molecular of covalent substances (*see* Chapter 5) do not conduct electricity because they contain no free electrons. For the same reason ionic compounds are non-conductors. However, when ionic substances—acids, bases, salts—are dissolved, they break up into ions which are free to move through the solution. Pure water is *not* a conductor, but when these substances are dissolved in it, the solution does conduct electricity by movement of these charged particles (ions). A solution which conducts electricity by the movement of its charged ions is known as an *electrolyte*.

In one important way the conduction of electricity by solutions differs from conduction by metals in that the former is attended by chemical change. This process of chemical change is called *electrolysis*. The process of electrolysis requires a supply of electric current, connected to two parts of a circuit (one attached to the negative pole and one to the positive pole of the current source) immersed in a solution (*see* Fig. 6.3).

The first quantitative studies of electrolysis were made by Michael Faraday in 1833. Much of his terminology is still used today. The two parts of the circuit which are in contact with the solution Faraday called 'electrodes'. The electrode connected to the positive pole he called the 'anode' and the one attached to the negative pole, the 'cathode'. Faraday also first introduced the word 'electrolyte'. Of the ions in solution, those which were attracted to the anode he called 'anions' and those attracted to the cathode he called 'cations'.

The apparatus (vessel, electrodes, electrolytes etc.) in which electrolysis is carried out is called an *electrolytic cell* or *voltameter* (the latter not to be confused with the voltmeter).

Industrial Applications of Electrolysis

One of the earliest industrial applications of the electric current was in the coating of base metals with a layer of a more expensive metal,

a process known as *electroplating*. The object to be coated is the cathode and the metal with which it is to be coated, the anode. The electrolyte must contain ions of the same metal as the anode in order that the metal can be transferred across to the cathode. In silver plating, for instance, the anode is of silver and the electrolyte a solution of a silver salt such as silver nitrate (*see Fig.* 6.3). The process of electrolysis is also used in the refining of metals.

The electrolysis of sodium chloride solution, which yields chlorine gas at the anode and sodium hydroxide in solution, is one of the main processes on which the giant alkali and chlorine industries were based. The manufacture of disinfectants, anaesthetics, insecticides, solvents, plastics and bleach are just a few of the industrial processes which use chlorine.

Electrolytes and Medicine

Of course the term 'electrolyte' is not relevant

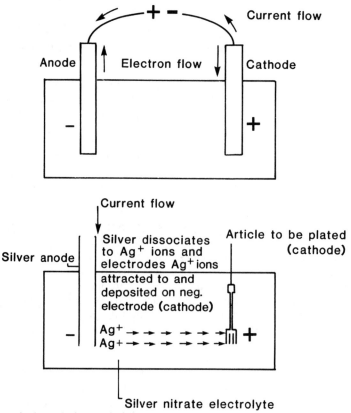

Fig. 6.3 Electrolysis and electroplating.

only to industrial processes. It is a word with which nurses will be familiar, for in human beings electrolytes are essential for the control of body fluids. For example, it is by excreting surplus inorganic ions that the kidney helps to maintain the body's electrolyte balance.

The electrolytes most essential to the maintenance of health are:

- Sodium chloride (NaCl)
- Potassium chloride (KCl)
- Sodium bicarbonate ($NaHCO_3$)
- Potassium bicarbonate ($KHCO_3$)

Other essential electrolytes are:

- Calcium chloride ($CaCl_2$)
- Calcium phosphate ($Ca_3[PO_4]_2$)
- Magnesium chloride ($MaCl_2$)

Electrophoresis

Electrophoresis, a means whereby substances can be separated because of their relative electro-negativity or electro-positivity, is another important use of electrolysis. For example, it is used in the laboratory for the separation of the different proteins contained in blood plasma. Plasma proteins, having a negative charge, move towards the anode. Because different proteins move at different speeds, it is possible to identify each type.

Conduction of Electricity through Gas

All gases, including air, are normally good insulators but they will conduct under special conditions. In all cases of conduction through a gas the charge is carried by ions and electrons.

Although a few molecules of gas in air are continually being ionized—by cosmic radiation from space, radiation from radioactive substances on the ground and by combustion in the atmosphere—the majority of molecules in a gas are normally neutral and the number of ions remains low because they soon recombine and become neutral again.

A very high voltage between electrodes can start conduction through a gas, as can an increase in the number of ions and free electrons present. The number of ionized gas molecules can be increased by exposing gas to ionizing radiations such as X-rays or alpha particles. Reducing the gas pressure of a sealed tube, such as a fluorescent tube, helps any free electrons to produce more ions and free electrons by collisions between gas molecules. Both high voltage and low gas pressure are used in fluorescent lamps and in gas discharge tubes such as those used for illuminated advertising signs. The colour of the sign is determined by the type of gas used.

Magnetism and Electric Currents

A magnet will set up a magnetic field in the same way that an electric charge sets up an electric field. In 1819 Hans Christian Oersted, a professor of physics at Copenhagen, discovered that an electric current in a wire produced a magnetic field. It is now known that a magnetic field will be created around all moving charges, whether or not they are in a wire.

The discovery of the connection between electricity and magnetism prompted other scientists, Faraday, Henry and others, to try to discover whether a magnetic field would generate a current of electricity. Faraday found that a current would only be produced by a *changing* magnetic field. An electric current will be induced in a loop of wire if the magnetic field in the loop is changing. This phenomenon, known as *electromagnetic induction*, is the basis of all our supplies of electricity. Any change in an electric field will produce changes in the magnetic field and vice versa *ad infinitum*. These changes give rise to electromagnetic waves (*see* Chapter 3).

7

Heat

Heat transforms solids into liquids, liquids into gases and gases into plasma. Heat is felt when the sun shines or when a fire burns. When a nail or metal sheet is hammered or a rope pulled through clenched hands heat is produced—examples of the way in which heat can be produced by mechanical energy. The process can of course be reversed. Heat can be used to produce mechanical energy and one example of this is the lifting of a kettle lid by the steam produced when water is boiled—a phenomenon which reputedly provided the inspiration for Watt's steam engine.

The Nature of Heat

For many centuries the effects of heat have been studied, but it was James Joule (1818–89) whose experiments, in 1842, discovered the true nature of heat. Joule converted measured amounts of mechanical energy and electrical energy into heat and found that the amount of heat produced was always proportional to the amount of energy used. Heat is thus the form in which energy is converted from one type to another.

The amount of heat contained in any body is the product of its mass, temperature and specific heat capacity.

Mass depends on the number and size of the atoms contained in the substance.

Temperature is a measure of 'hotness' of a substance and determines the rate at which heat will be transferred to or from a substance.

The *specific heat capacity* of any body is defined as the heat required to raise its temperature by 1 K (degree Kelvin). The amount of heat needed to raise the temperature of a substance depends on its nature as well as its mass. For example, if equal masses of water and oil are exposed to the same quantity of heat for the same period of time, the rise in oil temperature will be greater than that of the water. After 3 minutes exposed to a gas burner oil will rise 10 K whilst water will rise only 5 K. As the masses of both substances are equal and the supply of heat the same, it follows that oil has a smaller specific heat capacity than water.

Very few substances have a higher heat capacity than water; hydrogen is a notable exception and its high heat capacity together with its high thermal conductivity makes it an efficient cooling gas.

Latent Heat

The heat energy which changes the state of a substance—from solid to liquid, liquid to gas—is called *latent heat*. Much more energy is needed to turn boiling water into steam than to boil the water in the first place. Once boiling, the water temperature remains constant at 100 °C even though heat energy is still being added, the excess energy being used to convert the water from its liquid to its gaseous (vapour) state. This extra energy does not show its presence by a change in temperature. Latent heat is therefore concealed or hidden heat.

When steam condenses to form water, excess energy—latent heat—is given off. This is one reason why a scald from steam is more damaging than one from boiling water, for as the steam condenses excess energy in the form of latent heat is transferred to the tissues.

Evaporation

Evaporation causes cooling but requires heat energy. Molecules on the surface of a liquid can either escape to the atmosphere or fall back into the liquid. The faster-moving molecules, that is those with most energy, will escape. Those with less energy will remain in the liquid unless more heat is added, the average energy of the molecules in the liquid will be lowered, so the liquid itself will be cooler.

Some liquids, such as methylated spirits and ether, have low boiling points (are *volatile*) and so will change readily from liquid to vapour at room temperature. When such liquids come into contact with the skin they feel cold. This is because the body loses heat—energy—to the liquid; in other words, the liquid acquires latent heat from the body and vaporizes or evaporates.

Water and sweat evaporate from the skin in the same way, although, having somewhat higher boiling points than either methylated spirits or ether, the process takes longer and the cooling effect is not so immediately obvious. The application of cold water or methylated spirit to the skin are methods used therapeutically to increase the rate of heat loss by evaporation and so reduce the body temperature of febrile patients.

Transmission of Heat

Heat can be transmitted by conduction, convection and radiation.

Conduction

When one end of a metal rod is heated, the unheated end soon becomes warm. This is because heat travels through the metal by the process of *conduction*.

All electrons are constantly vibrating and in metals the electrons are mobile (*see* Chapter 5). When a metal is heated the kinetic energy of its electrons is increased and they begin to move more rapidly and to move towards the cooler parts of the metal. Here

their energy is transferred to the cooler molecules. At the same time cooler, and therefore slower-moving, electrons drift towards the heated end.

Energy is also transmitted through metals by the vibrations of the atoms themselves, although to a lesser extent. This energy is passed on in the form of high frequency waves in tiny energy packets called *phonons* (not to be confused with photons, *see* Chapter 3). In non-metals, which have no free electrons, energy is transmitted entirely by this process.

Thermal Conductivity

Thermal conductivity is a measure of the heat conducting property of a material. Most metals are good conductors—silver and copper being exceptionally good. Wood, glass, cork, cotton and wool are examples of bad conductors. Textiles are bad conductors of heat because their fibres enclose tiny pockets of air. Loss of body heat is minimized by a covering of poorly conducting material, i.e. clothing. All gases, including air, are poor conductors. Double glazing reduces heat loss because of the layer of poorly conducting air between the two panes of glass. Stone is a better conductor of heat than wool, hence a stone floor feels colder than a carpeted floor even at the same temperature because stone conducts heat *away from* the body more readily than a carpet.

It is the high thermal conductivity of metal which made possible the development of the miner's safety lamp—the Davey lamp. The flammable gas methane is often found in mines and when coal output was increased in the eighteenth century to meet the demands of new industries, explosions became commonplace. The first safety lamp was a simple oil burner totally surrounded by a cylinder of wire gauze. The wire conducts the heat away so rapidly that the air passing through the gauze is not hot enough to ignite the methane. The development of the safety lamp was one of the first occasions on which science was positively applied in the interest of safety.

With the exception of molten metals, liquids are poor conductors and gases are even worse. However, heat can rapidly be transmitted through liquid by the process of convection.

Convection

In the process of conduction heat is transferred from one part to another, for example from electron to electron or atom to atom. In the process of *convection* heat is carried by, and transferred by, the movement of a liquid or gas. When liquid is heated at the bottom of a container a current of hot liquid moves upwards to be replaced by a current of cold liquid moving down.

Liquid expands on heating so that when liquid near the bottom is heated, it becomes less dense and therefore will rise. If the liquid at the *top* of the vessel is heated it will expand and float on the denser cooler liquid beneath. The small amount of heat which might travel down will do so by conduction not convection. Warm air near a heat source, such as a fire or radiator, will be conducted to colder regions and be replaced by colder air. This in turn will be heated and so the process continues, with warm air rising and being replaced by colder air. In this way warmth can be transmitted to all parts of a room.

During the eighteenth century coal mines were ventilated by convection. Two shafts, the up-cast and the down-cast, were sunk and a fire lit at the bottom of the up-cast shaft heating the air and causing it to rise. Fresh air was consequently drawn down the down-cast shaft and passed through the mine passages. In turn this air became heated and drawn up through the up-cast shaft to be replaced by more fresh air via the down-cast shaft.

Natural convection also occurs in the air. Breezes and winds arise when air from a warm region moves to a colder neighbouring region.

Conduction and convection are methods of heat transfer which both require a medium. There is a third method of heat transfer which requires no medium.

Radiation

Radiation is the way in which heat travels from the sun across space to the earth's atmosphere. This 'radiant energy' consists of invisible electromagnetic waves which are partly reflected and partly absorbed. It comes from the sun either directly or indirectly, and when coming directly travels through 150 million km of space. Like light, which being part of the electromagnetic spectrum is fundamentally the same type of energy (*see* Chapter 3), it travels in a straight line.

Radiant heat is absorbed by all objects, although dull black and dark matt objects absorb heat more readily than bright light-coloured surfaces. (This is why light-coloured clothing is preferred in hot weather.) Radiant heat is also given off by all surfaces, and again black surfaces lose heat more readily than light ones.

Body Heat

The normal body temperature in man is generally stated to be about 37 °C (98 °F). Although this varies in different parts of the body (for instance oral temperature is slightly lower than rectal temperature), the central body, or core temperature, remains constant.

Because cells survive only within a narrow temperature range, it is necessary to maintain a constant body temperature even when external conditions (environment) and internal conditions (metabolism and muscular activity) vary. This is achieved by balancing the amount of heat lost against the amount gained. Several activities such as vasoconstriction, vasodilatation, sweating, muscle tone and shivering help to maintain the balance between heat loss and heat gain. The several centres which govern these activities are integrated by the hypothalamus which effectively 'sets' the body temperature.

Heat Gain

Heat is gained by metabolism. Without loss of heat normal metabolism would increase the body temperature by 1 °C every hour. To a lesser extent, heat is gained from a hot environment and from eating hot food and drinks.

Heat Loss

Heat is lost from the body via the skin, the lungs and excretions. The most important route of heat loss is via the skin. Depending on external and internal circumstances, about 85 per cent of heat loss occurs in this way. The average heat loss of the average male adult is equivalent to that of a 60 watt electric bulb. Heat is lost via the skin in the three ways of heat transmission already described, that is conduction, convection and radiation.

Conduction is usually the least important method. It occurs when the body comes into contact with colder objects, such as a cold floor. Convection occurs when warmed air currents coming from the body meet air of a lower temperature. Radiation also occurs when the ambient temperature is lower than the body temperature, heat passing from the body in the form of invisible infrared rays (*see* Chapter 3).

The body can also lose heat by the evaporation of water (sweat) from the skin. When the environmental temperature is higher than 37 °C, heat will be gained by the body rather than lost and then evaporation will be the only way in which the body can lose heat. Evaporation is a very efficient cooling method when the air is dry, but as humidity increases it becomes less effective.

Disturbances in Temperature Regulation
Hypothermia
If exposed to severe cold the body temperature may fall to below 35 °C (95 °F), when a state of *hypothermia* exists. Young babies and elderly people are particularly at risk. Hypothermia reduces the rate of metabolism and the supply of blood to the tissues, a fact which is used to advantage in some surgical procedures. Coma may occur, in which case metabolism is further reduced, movement ceases and the temperature drops more rapidly.

Heat Cramp
Heat cramp follows profuse sweating in an atmosphere of low humidity and high temperature. Dehydration can be prevented by the intake of fluids, but loss of salt (NaCl) will cause heat cramp. This can be avoided by the addition of 0.2 per cent saline to drinks.

Heat Stroke
Heat or sun stroke occurs in conditions of high temperature and high humidity, which prevent both radiation and evaporation. A failure of the body's heat regulating system ensues: sweating ceases, the skin becomes dry and hot, the temperature may rise to 43 °C (110 °F) and death may ensue.

Heat Exhaustion
Heat exhaustion occurs when the removal of metabolic heat from the body to the environment becomes difficult. The body responds to an increase in its temperature by increasing cardiovascular activity, increasing the pulse rate in order to pump more blood to the skin, so raising the skin temperature in relation to the temperature of its environment. When vasomotor control and cardiac output prove inadequate to meet the increased demand put upon them by increased vasodilatation, heat exhaustion is said to occur.

8

The physical states of matter

As previous chapters have discussed, all elements are composed of atoms. They exist in four different states or phases—solid, liquid, gas and plasma—all of which are interchangeable (see *Fig.* 8.1).

The physical properties of elements in their various phases can be explained in terms of the forces that exist between molecules. These forces arise out of the potential electrical energy (*see* Chapter 2) which exists between the molecules and the kinetic or thermal (heat) energy of the molecules themselves, which depends on the temperature of the substance. The particular state or phase of a substance, together with the properties which it then possesses, are determined by the relative magnitudes of these two energies.

Solids may be aggregates of either atoms or molecules. The forces which hold them together are electromagnetic in nature (*see* Chapter 6). When the centres of atoms are a certain distance apart, the attractive force between them is zero—the *zero force position*. When they come closer than this specific distance they repel and when further apart they attract one another. Even in a solid state molecules are constantly in motion, vibrating about their zero force positions, alternately attracting and repelling each other. However, molecules in their solid state do not possess enough energy to break free from their neighbours, even though as their temperature is increased they acquire greater kinetic energy which allows them to move further apart. This explains why solids are confined to a particular shape but expand when heated (i.e. when they are supplied with more thermal energy).

When sufficient energy (heat) is supplied, the substance will enter its liquid phase. Molecules in a liquid do possess enough energy to break their bonds with each other so are free to move at random within the substance. Given sufficient energy they can move past and around each other and change their position relative to each other. But there will remain some attraction between them and so individual particles will not be able to break free. Although the volume of any given amount of liquid will remain constant, the substance will no longer have a definite shape and will conform to the shape of its container (*see Fig.* 8.2).

Further energy (heat) input will be required to provide the particles with sufficient kinetic energy to overcome all the attractive forces between them. This is the gaseous phase in which mobile molecules have little or no interaction with each other. Although collisions between molecules will occur, they are free to move independently of each other. A gas has no definite volume and will expand to fill all available space (*Fig.* 8.2).

Heating gas to millions of degrees centigrade provides sufficient energy to allow electrons to break free from gas molecules which are therefore ionized. Ionized gas is now considered to be the fourth state of matter and is called *plasma (see below)*.

The transitions from solid to liquid, liquid to gas and gas to plasma are thus all dependent on a supply of energy (heat). The amount of energy necessary for the transition will vary considerably for different substances. For instance, most metals are solid at room

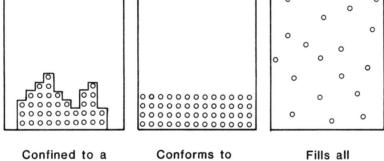

Fig. 8.1 The physical states of matter.

SOLIDS   **LIQUIDS**   **GASES**

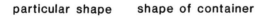
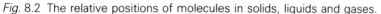

Confined to a   Conforms to   Fills all
particular shape   shape of container   available space

Fig. 8.2 The relative positions of molecules in solids, liquids and gases.

temperature—mercury being the exception—whilst other elements, such as hydrogen and oxygen, exist as gas at room temperature. Water readily converts from solid (ice) to liquid (water) to gas (steam).

When a substance changes its state its density changes also. An element in its solid state, where the atoms are closely bound, will have a higher density than the same element in liquid form, where the atoms are less closely bound and, in turn, the liquid form will have a higher density than the gaseous form, where atoms are free to move independently of each other. The densities of gases vary to a much greater extent with changes in temperature than do those of solids and liquids. For this reason it is necessary always to record both temperature and pressure when stating the densities of gases.

Plasma

Plasma occurs naturally in the interior of stars

(including the sun) and in the interstellar space of the Aurora Borealis (the Northern Lights). Plasma, now considered to be the fourth state of matter, is included here because of the scientific and industrial applications of matter in this state. As stated, plasma is produced by heating gas to tens of millions of degrees centigrade when a high percentage of the atoms will be ionized. This technique is used in attempts to release energy by fusion of elements of low mass to produce elements of greater mass. Heat from plasma is easily lost however and so the ions are short-lived. One of the major difficulties encountered in the course of thermonuclear experiments in the laboratory is to retain heat and so prevent the plasma reverting to a gas.

Plasma flame is used in industry to produce coatings of a quality unattainable by any other means. In this process, the rapid loss of heat is an advantage. Powder particles of the coating material, when introduced into the thermal plasma spray, will be melted and projected on to the object to be coated. Although the temperature of the plasma flame close to the nozzle outlet is high, heat dissipates so rapidly that the article being coated does not overheat (and neither, of course, does the operator). These coatings are used when heat, wear and corrosion resistance are essential, as for example in aero-engines, rockets and missiles.

Gases

In a gaseous state the average distance between particles and the average speed of vibration is much greater than in the liquid state. A gas has no definite shape or volume—it will expand to fill all available space. Gas molecules are in constant motion, and although there are no bonds between them, they will collide with each other and with the sides of their container. These collisions are responsible for the outward force (pressure) exerted by a gas on its container. (An inflated balloon retains its 'shape' because of the pressure exerted by the mobile gas molecules in collision with the inner surface of the balloon.) The speed of vibration of particles again depends on temperature; an increase in

temperature will cause the particles to move faster and so the force resulting from the collisions will increase. This is why the pressure of a given volume of gas will increase as the temperature is raised.

All gases, including those in solution such as bubbles in champagne or oxygen in blood, behave according to certain physical laws. Some understanding of the laws applicable to the properties of gas and the relationship between pressure, volume and temperature, is essential for an understanding of human physiology, i.e. inhalation and expiration of air, gas exchange, blood gases. The greater part of the potential energy of food (glucose, *see* Chapter 2) is liberated in the process of oxidation (*see* Chapter 5) and for this a continuous supply of oxygen is needed. The waste product of the oxidation of glucose is carbon dioxide gas and this must be removed. An exchange of gases between a human being, or any other living organism, is therefore essential. In man this process—pulmonary respiration—occurs in the lungs, where oxygen is transferred from air to the bloodstream and where carbon dioxide, together with some water, is eliminated from the bloodstream and passed to the environment. Appreciation of the properties of gases is also helpful for an understanding of industrial processes, including working in compressed air and methods of air purification, and of treatment methods used in hyperbaric medicine and cryosurgery.

The temperature, pressure and volume of any gas are properties which are interdependent. In order to study the relationship between them it is necessary to keep one of these factors constant (unchanged) while examining the other two.

Pressure and Volume

The expression 'Nature abhors a vacuum' has been attributed to Aristotle. We now know that outer space, which constitutes the greater part of the universe, is mostly a vacuum, but before the seventeenth century the abhorrent vacuum theory was held to be a valid scientific principle which was used to explain many phenomena. For instance, it was believed that water would rise when a pump was operated simply to prevent the creation of a vacuum. It was Robert Boyle (1627–91), experimenting with mercury, who proved that air pressure was the force responsible.

Boyle was the first scientist to investigate the relationship between the pressure and volume of a given mass of gas at a constant temperature. He used two J-shaped glass tubes which were closed at the short end. Mercury was then introduced into both tubes until the levels were the same on each side of the bend, leaving a quantity of air (which is a mixture of gases of course) in the short (enclosed) end. He found that increasing the amount of mercury to double the amount of pressure exerted on the trapped air, reduced the volume of air 50 per cent (*see Fig. 8.3*). Thus, at a constant temperature, if the pressure on a given mass of gas is halved, its volume will be doubled. Conversely, if the pressure is doubled the volume will be halved. This is the essence of *Boyle's Law*, which states:

The volume of a fixed mass of gas is inversely proportional to the pressure provided the temperature remains constant.

This can be expressed by the equation

$$p_1V_1 = p_2V_2 \text{ or } pV = \text{constant}$$

where p_1V_1 refers to one pair of values for a given mass of gas, and p_2V_2 the second pair for the same mass.

If a given mass of gas is placed in a container with a piston (such as a syringe) then the gas can be made to expand and contract (or its volume to increase or decrease) by moving the piston. Provided there is no increase or decrease in temperature, when the piston is depressed, the gas will be confined in a smaller space and its density and pressure on the sides of the vessel increased. Similarly, when the piston is released the gas will expand to fill the larger space, and its density and pressure will be reduced (*see Fig. 8.4*).

Volume and Temperature

The relationship between volume and temperature at a constant pressure was investigated by Jaques Charles (1746–1823). If the pressure of a given mass of gas is constant then it can be shown by experiment that the volume of a gas increases as its temperature rises. A graph of the results of such experiments proves to be a straight line, suggesting a 'linear relationship' between volume and temperature (*see*

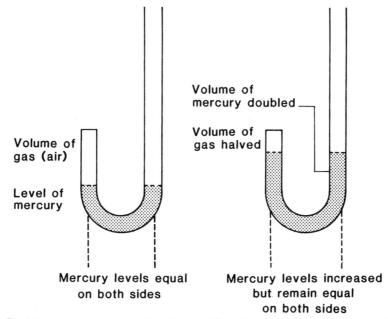

Fig. 8.3 Boyle's experiment showing the relationship between pressure and volume of a given mass of gas.

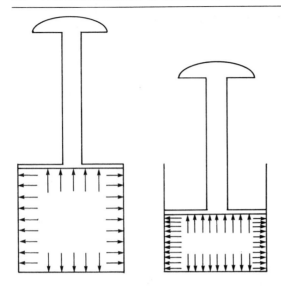

Fig. 8.4 Change of pressure with change of volume. Arrows indicate the direction of pressure exerted by gas molecules on the sides of the container.

Fig. 8.5). *Charles' Law* states:

The volume of a given mass of gas whose pressure is maintained constant is directly proportional to its absolute temperature.

This can be expressed as:

$$\frac{V}{T} = \text{constant}$$

where V = volume and T = temperature.

Charles found that raising the temperature of a gas from 0 °C to 1 °C produced an increase in pressure of 1/267 of the pressure at 0 °C. Later and more exact work has shown this fraction to be 1/273·15. The implication of Charles' law is thus that if a gas is coooled to −273.15 °C its volume will become zero. The name *absolute zero* is now given to this temperature and measurements on the absolute temperature scale are denoted by the symbol A (0 °C = 273.15 °A).

Lord Kelvin (1824–1907), working largely theoretically, calculated the lowest possible temperature that could be reached and his result agreed very closely with absolute zero. The absolute temperature scale is often referred to as the kelvin scale, symbol K.

If the graph of volume against temperature (*Fig.* 8.6) is extrapolated the line cuts the temperature axis at −273 °C (zero kelvin, 0 K) at which temperature the volume of gas would theoretically contract to zero. This assumption cannot, of course, be proved or disproved by experiment because gas liquefies before this temperature is reached.

Temperature and Pressure
When volume is constant, results of experiments on the third relationship between temperature and pressure plotted on a graph show a straight line passing through −273 °C (or 0 K). Thus the pressure of the gas is proportional to its temperature measured on the kelvin scale. This is expressed as the *Pressure Law*, which states:

The pressure of a fixed mass of gas is directly proportional to its absolute temperature provided the volume remains constant.

In other words, the pressure divided by the temperature is constant or:

$$\frac{p}{T} = \text{constant}$$

The Gas Equation
The three relations between pressure, volume and temperature

Charles Law V/T = constant
Boyles Law p = constant
Pressure Law p/T = constant

can be combined into one equation

The gas equation pV/t = constant.

This formula can be used to make calculations about pressures and volumes when all three quantities (p, V, T) are changing at the same time provided the mass of gas is constant. Thus

$$p_1V_1/T_1 = p_2V_2/T_2$$

Universal Gas Law
Understanding the relationship between pressure, volume and temperature (p, V, T,) of gas

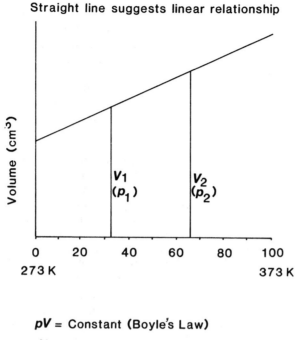

Straight line suggests linear relationship

$$pV = \text{Constant (Boyle's Law)}$$

$$\frac{V}{T} = \text{Constant (Charles' Law)}$$

$$\frac{P}{T} = \text{Constant (Pressure Law)}$$

$$\frac{pV}{T} = \text{Constant (includes all 3 laws)}$$

Fig. 8.5 The relationship between the volume and temperature of a gas at constant pressure.

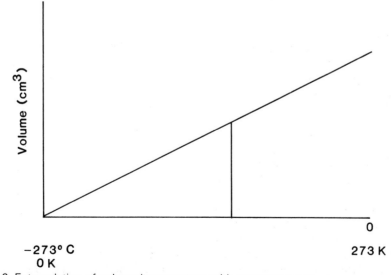

Fig. 8.6 Extrapolation of volume/temperature with constant pressure.

allows temperature to be defined by considering these properties. This is expressed by the equation

$$pV = RT$$

where p = pressure, V = volume, T = temperature and R = a constant. (For one mole of gas, R is a universal constant for all gases and has a value of 8.3 joules per degree kelvin.)

The law $pV = RT$ is called the *Universal Gas Law*. Many gases do not observe this law completely, but any gas which does obey the law precisely is called an *ideal gas*. In general all gases tend to behave as ideal gases as pressure decreases.

Partial Pressure

When a container, and in this case the human body constitutes a container, contains a mixture of gases, then the total pressure of the mixture is the sum of the pressures of all the individual gases when they have expanded to fill the container. Thus if a container holds 100 per cent oxygen it will exert a pressure of 760 mmHg (or one atmosphere); but if the same container holds a mixture of 20 per cent oxygen and 80 per cent nitrogen, it will still exert a pressure of 760 mmHg but of this 20 per cent (152 mmHg) will be exerted by the oxygen and 80 per cent (608 mmHg) by the nitrogen. The pressure of an individual gas in a mixture is called its *partial pressure* (p) or tension. It is the pressure which would be exerted if that gas alone occupied the same volume and had the same temperature as the mixture. This is *Dalton's Law of Partial Pressure* and can be expressed by the equation:

$$p_2 = h + H$$

or total pressure = partial pressure A plus partial pressure B.

Pulmonary Ventilation

A continuous supply of oxygen is essential to life. Pulmonary respiration, the exchange of oxygen and other gases between the environment and the individual, is governed by the gas laws.

The presure exerted on the rigid thoracic wall and the pressure existing in the lungs will be equal to atmospheric pressure which, for the purpose of this discussion, will be assumed to be normal, that is 760 mmHg. The

expiration and inspiration of normal breathing will be accompanied by an increase and decrease in air pressure in the lungs. The degree of pressure change depends on the rate and depth of breathing and on the amount of resistance encountered. During quiet breathing pressure changes will be in the region of 2–3 mmHg and during laboured breathing in the region of 5–10 mmHg. When the air passages are obstructed, pressure during inspiration can be reduced by 30–70 mmHg and during expiration, increased by 40–100 mmHg.

The volume of air entering and leaving the lungs during respiration, like the pressure of air in the lungs, will be determined by the rate and depth of breathing. During inspiration the volume of air in the lungs increases (as the pressure decreases) and decreases during expiration. Changes in volume of air in lungs can be observed as the circumference of the chest increases and decreases.

Because the lungs are elastic, they will collapse when removed from the body. When a lung is removed, a partial vacuum is created in the pleural cavity and the interpleural pressure will be reduced by about 5 mmHg to 755 mmHg. It is this negative intrapleural pressure which prevents further collapse of any remaining lung tissue.

Diffusion of Gases

Respiration depends on the diffusion of gases between the individual and the environment. Gases spread from an area of high pressure to one of low pressure and if several gases are present, as in air, the molecules of each gas will diffuse and exert pressure independently of each other. It is the pressure differentials which provide the force necessary to drive gases from one side of the respiratory membrane to the other.

Diffusion also takes place when gases are dissolved in liquid. The movement of gas molecules into and out of a liquid, that is the solubility of a gas, is governed by *Henry's Law*, which states:

The quantity of a gas dissolved is proportional to the partial pressure of the gas above the liquid.

This can be expressed mathematically as:

$$\frac{Vg}{Vl} = aP$$

Where Vg = volume of gas, Vl = volume of liquid and aP = the partial pressure of the gas.

Molecules of gas are in constant motion and those exposed to the surface of a liquid will be dissolved. Initially a large number of molecules will enter the liquid rapidly but almost immediately a few begin to leave. When the pressure of the gas outside the liquid equals that of the dissolved gas, the number entering will equal the number leaving, i.e. a state of equilibrium will exist. Reducing the gas pressure will upset this equilibrium and the number of molecules leaving will exceed the number entering until equilibrium has been restored.

The quantity of gas dissolved at a given temperature and pressure will depend on the nature of the gas and of the liquid. For example, under standard conditions (0 °C and 760 mmHg) 100 ml of water will take up 49 ml of oxygen and 171 ml of carbon dioxide, but at 40 °C the amount of both gases will be reduced, oxygen to 2·3 ml and carbon dioxide to 53 ml.

In the living body, the uptake and release of gases (for example oxygen and carbon dioxide) are governed by Henry's Law.

Blood is exposed to the pressure of air in the alveoli, not to atmospheric pressure. Thus 100 ml of water exposed to the pressure of air in the alveoli would take up about 0·33 ml of oxygen, but under the same conditions blood takes up 20 ml of oxygen, about 60 times as much. This is because gases are not only governed by physical laws, they are also capable of participating in chemical reactions. A large amount of the oxygen in the blood is held there in chemical combination with haemoglobin in the form of oxyhaemoglobin. The partial pressure of oxygen in blood is due to dissolved oxygen not to that chemically bound to haemoglobin.

The partial pressure of oxygen arriving at the lungs in the pulmonary capillaries is 40 mmHg which is less than the partial pressure of oxygen in the alveoli (100 mmHg), so oxygen will diffuse from the air into the blood. The greater partial pressure of oxygen in arterial blood than in either tissue fluid or cells forces the dissolved oxygen into the tissues and into the cells. (The resulting reduced partial pressure of oxygen in plasma forces the oxy-

haemoglobin to liberate its oxygen and this too passes from the plasma to tissues and cells.)

Changes in Atmospheric Pressure

Man is designed to breathe air (a mixture of gases) at a pressure of one atmosphere, when the partial pressures of the three main gases will be: oxygen 160 mmHg, nitrogen 596 mmHg and carbon dioxide 0·04 mmHg. At higher altitudes pressure will be reduced, whilst at depths below sea level it will be increased.

Small reductions in pressure occur as a result of increased altitude. Up to 10 000 feet, when the partial pressure of oxygen will be reduced to 110 mmHg, the body will become acclimatized on prolonged exposure. Aircraft are presurized to standard atmospheric pressure in order to avoid anoxia due to reduced partial pressure of oxygen.

Divers and those working in compressed air will be subjected to increased pressure. At only 33 feet the partial pressure of nitrogen will increase from 596 mmHg to 1192 mmHg. Because solubility of nitrogen, like any other gas, is governed by Henry's Law, the deeper a diver goes the greater will be the amount of nitrogen dissolved in the body fluids. If decompression to atmospheric pressure is too rapid, nitrogen will pass out of solution into the tissues. Nitrogen bubbles can occur anywhere in the body and may damage tissues or block small vessels with gas emboli—the condition called decompression sickness and commonly known as 'the bends' because of the acute pain caused by the presence of nitrogen bubbles in the tissues. By regulating the rate of ascent, decompression sickness can be prevented. For divers nitrogen can sometimes be replaced with another inert gas, such as helium.

Toxic Gases

One of the factors determining the toxicity of any substance is its physical state. The most direct route of entry to the bloodstream is via the lungs, so most substances in their gaseous state will gain entry this way more readily than in either the liquid or solid state, and will rapidly be carried around the body in the blood.

Gases which are toxic to humans can be

classified according to their mode of action as simple asphyxiants, chemical asphyxiants and irritant gases.

Simple Asphyxiants

Simple asphyxiants are physiologically inert. They do not undergo any chemical change, ill effects being caused when they are present in sufficient volume to reduce the partial pressure of essential oxygen. Nitrogen and carbon dioxide, which are normal constituents of air, fall into this category.

Chemical Asphyxiants

Chemical asphyxiants produce toxic effects through chemical reaction with metabolically important molecules. For instance, carbon monoxide is toxic because it combines with haemoglobin, which has an affinity for carbon monoxide 200 times greater than its affinity for oxygen. The compound formed, carboxy-haemoglobin, which is relatively stable, decreases the oxygen-carrying capacity of the blood. Carbon monoxide is a product of incomplete combustion and is found in mines, exhaust fumes from cars, fumes from furnaces, cigarette smoke etc.

Irritant Gases

Irritant gases such as ammonia, sulphur dioxide and chlorine, cause spasm of the glottis and so kill by strangulation. Because of their irritant nature the victim is more likely to be aware of their presence.

Liquids

In the liquid state atoms are free to move at random within the substance. This is because the atoms have acquired sufficient energy to allow them to move past and around each other and they can now change their position relative to each other. The higher the temperature, that is to say the more energy available, the faster will the atoms move, but there will still be some attraction (bonding) between them so individual particles will not be free to break away. Although a liquid has no definite shape, the volume of any given amount of liquid remains constant.

Surface Tension

It is possible to float a sewing needle on water by placing it first on filter paper on the surface of the water. The paper will absorb water and sink, leaving the needle floating. It will be found that the needle is resting in a slight depression as if the water were covered with an elastic skin. This property of liquid is known as the *surface tension*.

Although molecules can move freely through a liquid, the attractive and repulsive forces between them, which can vary according to the distance between molecules, can be just as strong as those in a solid. In the bulk of the liquid any particular molecule will be surrounded by an equal number of molecules on all sides; consequently the average distance between the molecules will be such that attractive and repulsive forces are equal. On the surface of the liquid, molecules are attracted downwards only. They pull together resulting in the elastic skin-like quality of the water. It is because of this surface tension that some insects are able to walk on water, liquids form spherical drops and soap forms spherical bubbles.

Surface tension will exist at any surface boundary of a liquid. For instance, the alveoli of the lungs are lined with water in which oxygen dissolves before it can diffuse through to the pulmonary capillaries. If too much air is expelled from the alveoli the sides will touch and a film of water will be formed. The surface tension of this water will hinder the passage of air and so additional respiratory effort will be needed to overcome this and to re-open the alveoli.

Capillary Action

There are two types of force which act upon liquid molecules. The attractive force between molecules of the same substance is called *cohesion* and the attractive force between molecules of different substances is called *adhesion*. Water will wet a glass surface because the adhesive forces between water molecules and glass are greater than the cohesive forces between water molecules. Waxing the glass will reduce the adhesive forces and the water will be pulled into spherical shapes. The cohesive forces between molecules of mercury are stronger than the adhesive forces between mercury and glass, which is why mercury will form spherical drops on glass.

When a narrow bore (capillary) tube is placed into any liquid capable of 'wetting', the greater adhesive forces between the liquid and the glass this will cause the liquid to rise in the tube to a height several centimetres above the height of the liquid by the phenomenon of capillary action. However, because of the greater cohesive forces between molecules of mercury, in the same circumstances mercury will sink below the height of the liquid; that is, it will cause a *capillary depression* (see *Fig.* 8.7).

Capillary action is responsible for the movement of blood through tissue capillaries. It also explains why oil rises up a lamp wick and why blotting paper is absorbent.

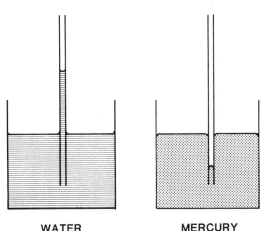

WATER	MERCURY
Adhesion of molecules for glass greater than their cohesion . Meniscus curves upwards and liquid rises in tube.	Cohesion of molecules greater than their adhesion for glass. Meniscus curves downwardsand is accompanied by a capillary depression

Fig. 8.7 Capillary action.

Viscosity
Any object moving through a liquid will meet resistance due to the frictional force (Chapter 2) of that liquid. The strength of this force is dependent upon the stickiness or *viscosity* of the liquid, which occurs as a result of the mutual atttraction of its molecules. In liquids such as water the frictional force, and therefore the viscosity, is relatively low. Liquids such as glue, glycerine and oil, having a relatively high resistance to flow and therefore a relatively high viscosity, are called *viscous fluids* (from the Latin *viscum*, 'made from mistletoe'). If a small object such as a ball bearing is allowed to fall through identical containers of different liquids it will fall more slowly through the liquid of higher viscosity.

Suspensions, Colloids and Crystalloids
Substances dispersed in liquid can be differentiated according to the size and behaviour of the particles.

Suspensions contain particles with a diameter greater than 0·0001 mm. They do not diffuse and can be separated by gravity or filtration. Blood, for instance, is a suspension of blood cells in plasma.

Colloidal solutions contain particles whose diameter lies between 0·0001 mm and 0·000 001 mm. These particles do not settle out by gravity but it is possible to separate them by rapid centrifugation. Colloids are large molecules or macromolecules of proteins and some polysaccharides (Chapters 11 and 12). Common examples of colloid solutions are starch, soap, gelatin and albumin. Proteins present in the living cell are in colloidal form.

In a true *crystalloid solution* the dispersed particles or crystalloids have a diameter of less than 0·0001 mm and these particles will be either ions or very small molecules. A true solution is homogeneous, there will be no settling out. Salts, acids and bases are true solutions (*see* Chapter 9).

Filtration
Materials in suspension or colloidal solution can be separated by filtration. This is a means whereby a force, such as gravity, or pressure, such as blood pressure, causes a substance in solution to pass through the pores of a membrane.

A membrane which allows the passage of a substance in this way is said to be 'permeable'. Permeability depends on the size of the molecule and the nature of the membrane. The size of pores will vary and membranes with very small pores, such as capillary walls, are called *ultrafilters*.

Crystalline solutions such as sugar or salt will diffuse more rapidly in water than will colloidal solutions such as albumin. This is because of the larger size of the albumin molecule. Any membrane which allows the passage of some but not all substances is said to be 'semi-permeable'.

Cellophane is a semi-permeable membrane which is used in the artificial kidney. By a process of dialysis the ions and small molecules of a true or crystalloid solution are separated from colloidal particles by using a dialysing membrane which is permeable to crystalloids but impermeable to colloids.

Biological membranes are 'selectively permeable', that is for any particular substance there will be a membrane to which it is permeable and another to which it is impermeable. It is this selective permeability which allows membranes to control and direct the movement of substances into and out of cells.

Diffusion

Diffusion occurs in liquids when the molecular concentration of a substance in solution is greater in one part of the liquid than another and when no barrier exists between them. Thus if a quantity of water is floated on top of a strong sugar solution the sugar molecules will diffuse into the water until they are evenly distributed throughout the solution.

The velocity of the molecules, or rate of diffusion, will vary according to the molecular weight of particles and the temperature of the solution.

Diffusion plays an important part in the transport both of materials from the blood to the cells and of cellular products to the blood.

Osmosis

When dried fruits such as prunes are soaked in cold water they more or less regain their original shape and size after a few hours. This is because water has passed through the cell walls of the fruit in a process called *osmosis*.

Osmosis is the passage of water, or any other solvent, through a selectively permeable membrane from a dilute to a more concentrated solution. For instance, if a strong salt or sugar solution is separated by a membrane from a large area of water, the water will pass into the solution. The movement of water (or solvent) will usually cause an obvious volume change but the movement of a solute has only a negligible effect. Dried fruit swells because the cells of the fruit contain a high concentration of sugar and are surrounded by a semi-permeable membrane.

Osmosis is important to the normal functioning of living things. For instance, it plays an important part in the excretion of waste products from the blood via the kidneys.

Osmotic pressure is the force which causes a solvent to move from an area of low concentration to one of high concentration. The average osmotic pressure of human blood is about 5100 mmHg or 6·7 atmospheres and is due chiefly to salts, sugar and waste products dissolved in plasma.

Solids

Solids may be aggregates of atoms of one element such as lead or diamonds, or of molecules of different elements, for example a rock such as granite which is a combination of different minerals.

Solids differ in appearance, consider for example a strand of wool and a lump of lead. They also differ in size from the very large to the very small. Dust is matter in its solid state even when particles are so small that they cannot be seen with the naked eye. If inhaled, dust will irritate the lungs and toxic substances which exist as dusts may, depending on the size of the particles, reach the alveoli of the lungs. Soluble particles can then be absorbed directly into the bloodstream and insoluble particles can damage lung tissue.

When a substance in its liquid state is cooled, it loses energy and so particles in the substance no longer move freely. Instead they pack closely together to form crystals or glasses.

Crystals

In *crystals* the atoms or molecules are packed fairly closely together in stable and regular three-dimensional arrays (the crystal lattice). The formation of this crystal lattice is dependent on the ability of molecules or atoms to move freely when in the liquid state. As the liquid cools they can move around until they find a suitable surface to which to attach themselves. In some crystalline solids the crystals produced are several centimetres in diameter. However, most are *polycrystallines*, which are agglomerates of small crystals (*crystallites*) of about 0·01–1·00 mm in diameter.

Glasses

If a substance in its liquid state is of a high viscosity the atoms or molecules may not be able to reach a regular position. Consequently in the resulting solid the molecular arrangement will be irregular and this is called a *glass*. Sandbased glasses are examples of this type of solid. Many plastics and ceramics consist of glassy and crystalline parts. Some crystalline substances can be transformed into glass, for example crystalline sugar can be converted to glass (toffee) by heating. *Fig.* 8.8 shows the

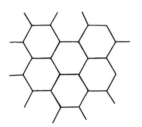

**a) Regular arrangement
of atoms in a crystal**

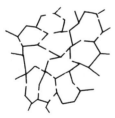

**b) Irregular arrangement
of atoms in glass**

Fig. 8.8 Arrangement of particles in (*a*) a crystal and (*b*) glass.

different arrangement of particles in crystal and glass.

The atoms in solids are held together by strong chemical bonds, and the type of bonding will determine such properties as hardness, malleability and brittleness (*see* Chapter 5). These bonds will require a large force to break them; consider, for instance, the strength needed to break an iron bar.

Although atoms in solids cannot alter their mean position relative to each other, they are in a constant state of motion or vibration. The speed of this vibration is dependent on the temperature of the solid, and as the temperature increases so does the speed of vibration. If more heat is added, some of this will be stored as heat energy, and some will be used to overcome the forces binding the atoms together. When this happens the atoms are free to move a little further apart.

This is how most substances expand when heated, although expansion of different substances heated to the same temperature will differ. For example, brass will expand more than steel and aluminium will expand more than brass. Glass has a smaller expansion than iron and Pyrex glass has a very low expansion. If there is any obstruction to the expansion of substances very large forces can be built up. This can cause problems in the construction of roads, buildings, bridges and machines, and design engineers have to make allowances accordingly. Positive use can also be made of the expansion of materials, for example in riveting. In order to get a tight joint a hot (expanded) rivet is inserted through the two plates to be joined and the end of the hot rivet hammered to form a second head. As it cools, the rivet contracts and pulls the two plates tightly together. The same process is used to fit steel tyres on to railway wheels and cartwheels.

When a solid is heated the extra energy provided makes the molecules vibrate more violently and push their neighbours further apart. If there is no room for expansion the molecules which make up the substance will, in trying to increase the space between themselves and their neighbours, produce the force which results in the expansion of the solid.

9

Ionic solutions

The concept of a solution was introduced in Chapter 8. Many familiar substances, including salt, sugar, soap, detergent, will dissolve in water. Other liquids, such as alcohol and trichlorethylene, also have the power to dissolve other substances. It is difficult to give a comprehensive definition of a solution, but it will be useful to examine the general process of the formation of a solution.

When a solid crystal of iodine is mixed with alcohol the crystal dissolves and the alcohol turns brown—the iodine is said to be *soluble* in alcohol. If a series of samples of this mixture are removed it will be found in all cases that the ratio of iodine to alcohol is the same. In other words, the mixture is uniform throughout; it is *homogeneous*.

When a quantity of carbon is mixed with alcohol, even when left undisturbed for a long period, as far as can be seen with the naked eye, the carbon does not dissolve and the alcohol does not change colour. If the carbon is distributed throughout the alcohol by stirring, it will settle out again when left undisturbed. This will be the case even when the carbon is in a very finely divided state, as in soot. Carbon is said to be *insoluble* in alcohol and the mixture is *inhomogeneous*.

A solution can therefore be defined as a homogeneous mixture of two or more substances. The substance which is dissolved is called the *solute* and the substance in which it is dissolved the *solvent* (solvent + solute = solution). When water is the solvent the solution is said to be an *aqueous solution*.

Solutions can be mixtures of solids, liquids or gases. When one liquid is dissolved in another, such as alcohol in water, the difference between solute and solvent may not be obvious. In such cases it is usual for the one which is present in larger volume to be called the solvent. Liquids such as water and alcohol which form a homogeneous mixture are said to be *miscible*. Liquids such as oil and water form an inhomogeneous mixture and are *immiscible*.

Solutions of solids in solids can also occur; these are important in geology but will not be considered further here.

Concentration
If more iodine is added to a solution of iodine in alcohol, this too will dissolve and the intensity of the colour of the liquid will intensify. In other words the *concentration*, or ratio of the weight of iodine to the weight of alcohol, has increased. This ratio—grammes of solute per 100 grammes of solvent—is a convenient measure of concentration and one with which nurses will be familiar. However, a better measure is the *molarity* of the solution. Molarity means the number of moles of solute in one litre of the solution. This unit is given as mol/l or sometimes is denoted by a capital M (*see* Appendix 3).

Saturation
If more crystals of iodine are added to the solution, the point will eventually be reached when the solid crystals cease to dissolve. If such a solution is maintained at a constant temperature and evaporation prevented (in other words if the system is closed) then the solid particles will settle at the bottom of the solution and the concentration of iodine will

remain unchanged. Any solution maintained at a constant temperature which contains a concentration of solute that cannot be exceeded at that temperature is said to be *saturated*.

Solubility
The concentration of a solution in a saturated solution is called its *solubility*. As with concentration, solubility can be expressed in terms of the number of grammes of solute per 100 g of solvent or by stating molarity. The constant temperature is important because solubility varies with changing temperature. Increasing temperature will increase the solubility of most solids. However, in a few instances, for example calcium sulphate ($CaSO_4$), an increase in temperature will result in decreased solubility.

Equilibrium
A saturated solution of iodine in alcohol is an example of *chemical equilibrium* (see Appendix 6). The solution will continue in equilibrium as long as it is kept in a sealed container at constant temperature.

Classification of Solutions
Chemists have for centuries been preoccupied with the classification of solutions, or of the solutes which form them. Early chemists showed a disrespect for the substances they were working with which would horrify any occupational health nurse today. Their practice of determining the characteristics of a substance by tasting or touching would be unthinkable today. However, through their foolhardiness, they noted that some substances had a sour taste, whilst others tasted bitter and were greasy to touch. Any substance with a sour taste they called an *acid* (Latin *acidus*, 'sour'). Substances that had a bitter taste and felt greasy they found could be obtained from the ashes of plants. These they called *alkalis* (Arabic *al qaliy*, 'heated ashes'). Subsequent work identified distinctive properties of acids and alkalis other than those noted by the early chemists.

Properties of Acids
- They are sour to taste, for example citric acid (citrus fruits) and acetic acid (vinegar).
- They are capable of changing the colour of indicators. (Indicators are dyes whose colour responds to the action of acids or alkalis: *Table* 9.1 shows how some indicators change.)

Table 9.1 The colour changes of some indicators

Indicator	Colour change acid	Colour change alkali
Methyl orange	Orange	Yellow
Methyl red	Red	Yellow
Litmus	Red	Blue
Phenolphthalein	Colourless	Red

- Many dissolve chalk (calcium carbonate $CaCO_3$) and metals such as zinc and copper with effervescence (the production of gas bubbles). When calcium carbonate dissolves the gas produced is carbon dioxide, and that produced when metals dissolve is hydrogen.
- They will damage living tissue. Weak acid will cause irritant dermatitis depending on the length of exposure. Individual susceptibility will vary, but if exposure continues anybody exposed will eventually be affected. Stronger acids will burn the skin and underlying tissues and some, such as chromic acid, will cause ulceration. Hydrofluoric acid is particularly hazardous, it will cause severe burning, erosion and ulceration. *Table* 9.2 lists some familiar acids.

Table 9.2 Some common acids

Acetic acid (vinegar)
Citric acid (citrus fruits)
Hydrochloric acid
Nitric acid
Tannic acid (tea)
Carbon dioxide

Properties of Alkalis
- They are bitter to taste and slippery to touch. Unlike acids, there are no familiar examples of commonly ingested alkalis! Soap and sodium carbonate (washing soda) are familiar examples that illustrate the slippery property of alkalis.

- They change the colour of indicators (*see Table* 9.1).
- All alkalis except ammonia will react with ammonium compounds to produce ammonia gas. Many cleaners contain alkalis such as ammonia or sodium hydroxide (caustic soda). Different types of cleaner must never be mixed because their constituent chemicals may react together to produce a toxic gas.
- Alkalis will damage living tissue. Weak alkalis will irritate the skin of any persons exposed, as will weak acids. Stronger alkalis, such as sodium hydroxide (caustic soda), will, as their common names imply, cause severe burning and deep-seated persistent ulcers. *Table* 9.3 lists some common alkalis.

Table 9.3 Some common alkalis

Sodium carbonate (washing soda)
Sodium hydroxide (caustic soda)
Potassium hydroxide (caustic potash)
Calcium hydroxide (caustic lime)
Ammonia

Neutralization
The distinctive properties of acids and alkalis disappear when one is added to the other. This type of reaction is called *neutralization*.

If, for example, hydrochloric acid is added to a solution of sodium hydroxide and the resultant solution allowed to 'dry out', that is if the water is allowed to evaporate, a white solid will remain. This tastes neither bitter nor sour; it is in fact sodium chloride ($NaCl$), common salt. The name *salt* is applied to the solid residue which is left following any neutralization reaction between an alkali and an acid. The general equation for this reaction is:

$$acid + alkali \rightarrow salt + water$$

Thus the chemical equation for the reaction between carbon dioxide (CO_2) and sodium hydroxide ($2NaOH$) to produce sodium carbonate (Na_2CO_3) and water (H_2O) would read:

$$2NaOH + CO_2 \rightarrow Na_2CO_3 + H_2O$$

If the water is allowed to evaporate a residue of sodium carbonate will remain.

Sodium carbonate is both a salt and an alkali. The three classes, acids, alkalis and salts, are therefore not mutually exclusive. Furthermore in some neutralization reactions there will be products other than salts and water. For instance, in the reaction between hydrochloric acid (HCl) and sodium carbonate ($NaCO_3$) bubbles of gas—carbon dioxide (CO_2)—will be produced, as the following equation shows:

$$Na_2CO_3 + 2HCl \rightarrow 2NaCl + CO_2 + H_2$$

Solutions at Molecular Level
The classification of solutions into acids, alkalis and salts according to their observed characteristics therefore gives no definite division between them. Neither does it explain why an acid or an alkali should possess specific properties. However, a study of reactions at molecular level will provide an explanation.

Bases
Experiments carried out at the beginning of the nineteenth century by the French chemist Lavoisier showed that oxides of lead (PbO) and oxides of mercury (HgO), although not soluble in water (and therefore it was not possible to test for acidity or alkalinity) did neutralize acids. In this sense, therefore, they possessed an alkaline quality and the word *base* was introduced to take account of this observation.

A base can be defined as any substance that can neutralize an acid. In other words it is a substance that reacts with an acid to form a salt. Bases include many insoluble metal oxides and hydroxides as well as alkalis.

The Molecular Formula of Acids
Lavoisier was convinced that oxygen was the vital element present in all acids. However, in 1810, Sir Humphrey Davey showed that hydrogen chloride, which is definitely an acid, contained no oxygen. It was the German chemist Liebig who, in 1838, suggested an acid to be a compound containing hydrogen which can be replaced by metals.

According to Liebig's definition, acids are made up of two parts; the hydrogen atoms which can be replaced by a metal, and another part called the *acid radical*. So hydrochloric acid (HCl) contains one replaceable hydrogen atom and the acid radical Cl. Sulphuric acid (H_2SO_4) contains two replaceable hydrogen atoms and the acid radical SO_4. Orthophosphoric acid (H_3PO_4) contains three replaceable hydrogen atoms and the acid radical PO_4. According to this theory, the number of hydrogen atoms an acid possesses indicates its basicity.

However, not all the hydrogen atoms contained in an acid are replaceable. For instance, the compound hypophosphorus acid (H_3PO_2) is 'monobasic', despite the fact that it contains three hydrogen atoms: i.e. in a neutralization reaction only one mole of sodium hydroxide per mole of hypophosphorous acid is produced.

$$NaOH + H_3PO_2 \rightarrow NaH_2PO_2 + H_2O$$

Theories based on Liebig's definition related acidity to molecular formulae but failed to explain why some hydrogen atoms are replaced and others are not. Neither did they suggest a molecular formula relevant to bases. These explanations can be found by examining what happens to solutes in solution.

Dissociation
Acid substances, when dissolved in water, *dissociate* (split up) into ions and exhibit a common factor, namely the formation of hydrogen ions (H^+). For example:

$$\text{hydrochloric acid } HCl \rightarrow H^+ + Cl^-$$

$$\text{nitric acid } HNO_3 \rightarrow H^+ + NO_3^-$$

$$\text{sulphuric acid } H_2SO_4 \rightarrow H^+ + SO_4^-$$

Bases dissolved in water also dissociate to form ions but the common factor they exhibit is the formation of hydroxyl (OH^-) ions.

$$NaOH \rightarrow OH^- + Na^+$$

Acids can therefore be defined as *substances that dissociate to form hydrogen (H^+) ions*. All non-metal oxides, for example carbon dioxide, sulphur dioxide, nitrogen dioxide, are acidic. An acid will be produced whenever a non-metal, such as carbon, is dissolved in water. In this instance the acid formed is carbonic acid.

Bases are defined as *substances that dissociate to form hydroxyl (OH^-) ions*. The commoner bases are ammonia, metal oxides and metal hydroxides.

An alkali is any base dissolved in water. Thus, all alkalis are bases and will react with acids to form salts. The most commonly used alkali is sodium hydroxide which will react with hydrochloric acid to form sodium chloride (common salt).

A salt is usually regarded as a compound produced by the replacement of the hydrogen ion of an acid by a metal. Each acid produces its own family of salts when it reacts with different bases: for example, hydrochloric acid will produce chlorides, e.g. sodium chloride; sulphuric acid will produce sulphides, e.g. magnesium sulphate; nitric acid will produce nitrides, e.g. ammonium nitrate. Sodium chloride and magnesium sulphate are examples of naturally occurring salts. Others, such as nitrites and sulphates needed for fertilizers, are produced by neutralizing acids commercially. Ammonium nitrate, an important fertilizer, is made by neutralizing nitric acid with ammonia:

$$HNO_3(aq) + NH_3(aq) \rightarrow NH_4NO_3(aq)$$

The water is evaporated leaving molten ammonium nitrate which is cooled into usable pellets.

Measuring Acidity
The acidity of a solution can be measured by determining the concentration of hydrogen ions in the solution. Highest concentrations are found in concentrated solutions of acids, such as hydrochloric (HCl), sulphuric (H_2SO_4) and nitric (HNO_3). Because of the wide range of possible concentrations a convenient scale—the pH scale—has been devised using the formula:

$$ph = -\log_{10}(H^+)$$

where H^+ = mole per litre in the solution.

Hydrogen (H^+) ions and hydroxyl (OH^-) ions may both be present in a solution, but an acidic solution will have the greater concentration of hydrogen ions, whilst the basic solution will contain the greater number of hydroxyl ions. To be neutral, designated pH7, there must be equal concentrations of hydrogen and hydroxyl ions in the solution. *Fig.* 9.1 shows the corresponding pH of various hydrogen ion concentrations. The scale ranges from 1 (a strong acid) to 14 (a strong base).

pH and the Living Organism

Living organisms can only tolerate a narrow range of hydrogen ion concentration. Human blood, for instance, must be close to pH 7·4 if life is to be maintained. If tissue pH falls below 7·3 acidosis occurs which can lead to coma and death. An increase in the tissue pH above 7·5 will result in alkalosis which can be the cause of convulsions and may also prove fatal.

Many industrial processes are critically influenced by changes in the pH of raw materials.

Buffer Solutions

A buffer solution is one in which the hydrogen ion concentration, and hence the acidity or alkalinity, is virtually unchanged by dilution.

The pH of a buffer solution will not change appreciably even if contaminated with traces of acid or alkali. An acidic buffer is prepared by mixing together precise quantities of a weak acid and the sodium or potassium salt of the same acid: for example, ethanoic acid and sodium ethanoate. Similarly an alkaline buffer is prepared by mixing a weak base and a soluble base of that salt: for example, ammonia solution and ammonium chloride. Solutions of weak or poorly ionized acid and its almost completely dissociated salt can prevent or at least minimize a drastic change in pH because the hydrogen ion concentration of such an acid/salt mixture will be considerably less than that of the acid itself.

Buffers can be regarded as regulators of pH by their ability to 'mop up' hydrogen and hydroxyl ions. The residue of metabolically produced acids which are not neutralized by bases taken in the diet is neutralized by the buffer systems of the body.

Keeping the pH of the body within its normal range is important because the behaviour of proteins varies greatly with changes of pH, and enzymes, which catalyse biochemical reactions, are highly specialized proteins acutely sensitive to changes in pH. The ratio of

	$[H^+]$ (mol/l)	pH
	1 or 10^0	0
	0.1 or 10^{-1}	1
	0.01 or 10^{-2}	2
Increasing	0.001 or 10^{-3}	3
acidity	0.0 001 or 10^{-4}	4
	0.00 001 or 10^{-5}	5
	0.000 001 or 10^{-6}	6
Pure water	0.0 000 001 or 10^{-7}	7
	0.00 000 001 or 10^{-8}	8
	0.000 000 001 or 10^{-9}	9
Increasing	0.0 000 000 001 or 10^{-10}	10
alkalinity	0.00 000 000 001 or 10^{-11}	11
	0.000 000 000 001 or 10^{-12}	12
	0.0 000 000 000 001 or 10^{-13}	13
	0.00 000 000 000 001 or 10^{-14}	14

Fig. 9.1 The range of hydrogen ion concentrations—the pH scale.

buffer systems in the body is known as the *acid base balance*.

The body is constantly producing acids, for example sulphuric acid and phosphoric acid from the oxidation of proteins, lactic acid from muscle activity, and carbonic acid from the combination of carbon dioxide, which is present throughout the body, and water:

$$CO_2 + H_2O \rightarrow H_2CO_3$$

The reaction of carbonic acid with haemoglobin in the red cells gives rise to the formation of positive hydrogen ions and negative bicarbonate ions:

$$H_2CO_3 \rightarrow H^+ + HCO_3^-$$

In the cell the negative bicarbonate ions combine with positive potassium ions to form potassium bicarbonate ($KHCO_3$), and in plasma they combine with positive sodium ions to form sodium bicarbonate ($NaHCO_3$).

In blood the ratio of bicarbonate to carbonic acid is $20:1$ and this represents a pH of 7.4. The bicarbonate–carbonic acid buffer system plays a key role in the regulation of the body's pH. However, its effectiveness is dependent on the ability of the respiratory system and the renal system to stabilize the constituent bases and acids. The carbonic acid concentration is regulated by the respiratory system and the bicarbonate concentration by the kidneys.

The Role of the Respiratory System

About 50 per cent of metabolically produced acids are neutralized by bases available in the diet. Excess acid (for example the sulphuric acid formed by the oxidation of proteins) is neutralized by sodium bicarbonate to form sodium sulphate, carbon dioxide and water. By increasing the concentration of carbon dioxide in the blood, the sodium bicarbonate–carbonic acid ratio is reduced, the blood becomes more acidic and the pH is lowered. The decreased pH stimulates the respiratory centre in the medulla and breathing increases, flushing out carbon dioxide via the lungs. Thus the acidity of blood is decreased and pH increased to normal levels. Blood pH levels above normal will produce depression of the respiratory centre until the level of carbon dioxide in the blood again returns to normal. A blood pH of over 7.8 causes tetany and stimulates the excretion of alkaline salts by the kidney.

The quantity of volatile acid in the form of CO_2 excreted by the lungs is far greater than that of any other acid eliminated from the body. By responding rapidly to changes in the pH of the blood, the respiratory system does not lower the concentration of the valuable bases sodium and potassium.

The Role of the Renal System

The kidney excretes acid in the form of the salts of sulphur and phosphates. Neutral salts are converted to acid salts and this increases the acidity of the urine. The kidney cannot produce urine with a pH lower than 4.4 and so excretion of acid in a free form, as in respiration, is severely limited. The kidney excretes acid salts of sulphates and phosphates and conserves bases by acidification of urine and by ammonia synthesis. Urine is acidified when a neutral salt, for example phosphoric acid (Na_2HPO_4), exchanges its sodium (Na) ions for hydrogen (H) ions and is excreted as an acid while sodium bicarbonate is reabsorbed into the bloodstream.

Strong acids, such as hydrochloric acid (HCl), are buffered in the blood by bicarbonate ions to form the neutral salt sodium chloride (NaCl). The sodium ions are exchanged for hydrogen ions, which combine with ammonia produced by the kidneys, and are excreted as ammonium chloride (NH_4Cl). The sodium ions combine with bicarbonate ions and are returned to the bloodstream. In this way the amount of sodium excreted is reduced and valuable bases are preserved. If the kidney loses the ability to produce ammonia, as in some kidney diseases, the acids in the bloodstream will not be adequately neutralized and acidosis will result.

General Applications

Acids, bases and salts are of importance because of their biological and industrial significance. Nurses will be familiar with the salts that are important to normal bodily function. These include calcium phosphate, which is present in bones, and calcium gluconate, potassium chloride and sodium chloride, all important for electrolyte balance. Other familiar salts include aluminium phosphate, an antacid powder, barium sulphate, used for barium meal X-rays, and magnesium sulphate, used as a purgative and as a paste for boils.

Acids are used in many industrial processes including the manufacture of explosives, fertilizers, paper, plastics and drugs. A country's industrial capacity might well be gauged by its annual consumption of sulphuric acid! Alkalis are also important for industry, for instance the manufacture of soap and rayon.

Salts provide raw materials for many products, including many medicines.

Alkaloids are a group of basic organic substances of plant origin which can react with acids to form salts. Each molecule contains at least one nitrogen atom in a ring structure. Alkaloids have been used as medicines since early times—quinine, atropine, nicotine, cocaine, ergotamine, digoxin, hyoscine and scopalomine are some familiar examples. Many are addictive, for example cocaine and morphine, and their use is controlled by legislation (Medicines Act 1968).

10

Metals

Of the 105 elements known to man, 84 are metals. The two elements silicon and oxygen make up 75 per cent of the earth's crust and metals make up most of the remaining 25 per cent. Since ancient times man has made use of metals for adornment and to make tools and equipment. Modern technology has made possible more sophisticated use of metals, but some metals can be harmful to man and the toxic metals have become a recognized occupational hazard. Some metals, such as sodium, potassium and iron, are normally found in the human body and are essential for life. Traces of others, such as cobalt, copper and magnesium, are only found in small amounts but are nevertheless essential. These are known as *trace elements*. Excessive quantities of some of these can be toxic. *Table* 10.1 shows the approximate amounts of metals which will be found in an average adult.

Table 10.1 Metals normally present in the human body

Calcium	1500 g
Potassium	150 g
Sodium	100 g
Magnesium	20 g
Iron	4 g
Zinc	2 g

traces of:
copper
aluminium
molybdenum
cobalt
manganese

The Properties of Metals
Some physical and chemical properties are *generally* typical of all metals.

Physical Properties
- They are malleable (can be hammered into shape) and ductile (can be drawn into wires).
- Most are very strong and can support heavy loads.
- They shine with a lustre.
- Many are sonorous, they 'ring' when struck.
- In their solid state they are good conductors of electricity.

With the exception of mercury, they are solid at room temperature and most have high melting and boiling points; copper, for example, has a melting point of 1083 °C. The alkali metals (Group 1 of the Periodic Table, *see* Chapter 4) are exceptions and have low melting points.

Chemical Properties
- They react with oxygen to form oxides, for example:

magnesium + oxygen → magnesium oxide
$$Mg \quad + \quad O \quad \rightarrow \quad MgO$$

Metal oxides are bases (*see* Chapter 9) (they react with acids to form salts). When the metal is ionized the ions are always positively charged (*see* Fig. 10.1).

Not all metals are typical, however. Sodium, for example, has a low melting point (98 °C), is so light it will float on water and so

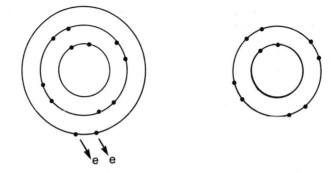

Magnesium atom − 2 electrons = magnesium^{++}ion

Fig. 10.1 The ionization of the magnesium atom.

soft it can easily be cut with a knife. Even amongst the typical elements no two will share exactly the same properties. The variations arise because of differences in their electronic structure.

Metallic Bonding
The atoms in a metal are closely packed in a strongly bound lattice. The outer valency electrons (those in the outer shell) break free of the parent atom to occupy or move through the spaces between the ions. Metals have been described as 'a lattice of ions in a sea of electrons'. This type of bonding explains why metals are malleable, ductile and good conductors of electricity.

Group I and II Elements
All the elements in Groups I and II of the Periodic Table are metals (see *Table* 10.2).

Table 10.2 Grouping of metals in the Periodic Table of the Elements

Group I	Group II
Lithium (Li)	Beryllium (Be)
Sodium (Na)	Magnesium (Mg)
Potassium (K)	Calcium (Ca)
Rubidium (Rb)	Strontium (St)
Caesium (Cs)	Barium (Ba)
Frankium (Fr)	Radium (Ra)

Group I elements, the alkali metals, show an oxidation state of +1, corresponding to the loss of one electron, whilst Group II elements (the alkaline earth metals), which contain two electrons in their outermost shell, have an oxidation state of +2. In both groups the chemical reactivity increases down the group, and this can be seen in reactions with cold water.

Lithium reacts slowly to produce lithium hydroxide and hydrogen gas:

$$2Li + 2H_2O \rightarrow 2LiOH(aq) + H_2$$

Potassium, further down the group, reacts rapidly with cold water and the hydrogen gas formed ignites spontaneously.

$$2K + 2H_2O \rightarrow 2KOH(aq) + H_2$$

Group II elements are less reactive; for example beryllium, at the top of the group, does not react at all with water and magnesium reacts only slowly with hot water, although rapidly with steam:

$$Mg + H_2O(g) \rightarrow MgO + H_2(g)$$

Further down the group calcium, like barium and strontium, does react with cold water:

$$Ca + 2H_2O \rightarrow Ca(OH)_2(aq) + H_2$$

Both the alkali and the alkaline earth metals react with chlorine to form chlorides and with oxygen to form oxides. For oxides the alkali metals conform to the general formula M_2O (M = metal), but the more reactive metals also form additional oxides called *peroxides* and *superperoxides* (*Table* 10.3).

All of the alkaline earth metals form typical oxides with the formula MO. Strontium and barium also form peroxides—StO_2, BaO_2.

Oxides of alkali metals react rapidly in water to form strongly alkaline solutions, such as sodium hydroxide ($2NaOH$). However, the tendency for alkaline earth metals to form alkaline solutions is less, although the alkalinity of solutions of both groups in water increases down the group.

Table 10.3 The metal oxides, peroxides and super-peroxides

Element	Oxide	Peroxide	Superperoxide
Lithium	Li_2O		
Sodium	Na_2O	(Na_2O_2)	
Potassium	K_2O	(K_2O_2)	(KO_2)

The chlorides of both groups are usually white crystalline ionic solids with high melting and boiling points. They are poor conductors of electricity in their solid state, but the ionic crystal lattices can be broken by melting or by dissolving in water and when molten or in solution they do conduct electricity. Beryllium chloride however is still a poor conductor of electricity even when molten. It is not soluble in water although it is soluble in organic solvents. This is because beryllium is more 'electronegative' than other elements in the group and so electrons cannot escape readily. This is why this metal shows a greater tendency to form covalent compounds (*see* Chapter 5).

Salts of Group I metals are generally soluble in water and form alkaline solutions. Salts of Group II metals, which contain ions with a 2^- charge, are generally less soluble.

The Transition Elements
The transition elements are a series of metals positioned in the Periodic Table between Groups II and III. Contained in this group are the more familiar metals. From scandium to zinc they are all silvery (except copper) and with the exception of zinc all have high densities and melting points.

These metals are much less reactive than either the alkali or the alkaline earth metals. However they do have some character-istic properties, including the formation of compounds in a wide variety of oxidation states (Chapter 5); copper, for example, has two common oxidation states—+1 (copper I) and +2 (copper II). This explains their catalytic properties. They form coloured compounds as the light of a certain colour is removed when electrons move from one orbital to another: for example, hydrated copper(II) ions absorb red light when electrons move and the residual blue light is transmitted to give hydrated copper(II) compounds their characteristic colour.

Ions of metals of this group which contain unpaired electrons show *paramagnetism*, that is, the production of a small magnetic field by the movement of such unpaired electrons. An extreme case of paramagnetism is *ferromagnetism*, a ferromagnet substance being one which has a permanent magnetic field.

Because atoms of the transition metals are similar in size and chemical nature they readily form alloys, for example brass, an alloy of copper and zinc. Alloys are usually harder, less malleable and have lower melting points than pure metals and will resist wear longer.

These metals also form *interstitial* compounds with carbon and hydrogen in which the small atoms of carbon or hydrogen fit into the spaces in the lattice of transition metals. Steel is such a compound, in which carbon atoms fit into the spaces between the iron lattice.

Metals of Other Groups
From Group III of the Periodic Table onwards the number of metals in each group decreases. Group V shows the transition from non-metal to metal down the group more clearly than any other group. Carbon and silicon are non-metals, germanium has properties between metal and non-metal and is called a *metalloid*, while tin and lead are metals (*see Table* 10.4).

Table 10.4 Elements of Group V

Carbon (C)	non-metal
Silicon (Si)	non-metal
Germanium (Ge)	metalloid
Tin (Sn)	metal
Lead (Pb)	metal

The Relative Reactivity of Metals

The reactivity of metals varies both within and between groups. Some react more vigorously than others; for example sodium will burn with oxygen with the application of only a little heat, iron will merely glow and give off sparks when heated to a high temperature, whilst gold will not react (burn) at all at any temperature. Similarly metals differ in their reaction with water. Potassium reacts violently with cold water whilst calcium reacts less vigorously and copper and gold do not react at all. In hydrochloric acid magnesium reacts vigorously, iron slowly, copper and gold not at all.

Acid is used by goldsmiths to test the purity of gold—the origin of the term 'acid test' applied to any decisive or searching test. The pattern followed by metals in their relative reactivity is called the *activity series*. Table 10.5 lists metals in descending order of reactivity.

Table 10.5 Activity series of some metals

Potassium (K)
Sodium (Na)
Magnesium (Mg)
Aluminium (Al)
Zinc (Zn)
Iron (Fe)
Lead (Pb)
Copper (Cu)
Silver (Ag)
Gold (Au)

Ancient and Modern Metals

The date of discovery of a particular metal gives some indication of its reactivity. The ancient metals, gold and silver, were used by earliest civilizations. Being unreactive they are found in the earth's surface in their pure state and so need no refining. More reactive metals are found in the form of chemical compounds or ores. Later civilizations learned to extract these metals by heating with carbon, hence the so-called Iron and Bronze Ages. Zinc, the most reactive of these ancient metals, was more difficult to extract and was not used until around the beginning of the Christian era.

Because it is so reactive, refining remained a difficult and expensive process until the twentieth century.

The 'modern metals'—aluminium, magnesium, sodium, potassium etc.—were unknown in their pure state two centuries ago. Being so reactive they cannot be extracted by heating. It was the discovery of electricity in the nineteenth century that made possible the extraction of these metals by electrolysis (*see* Chapter 6).

Because some metals are more reactive than others they 'compete' in chemical reactions. For example, when a mixture of iron and copper compete for oxygen, iron will always win to produce iron oxide. For the same reason iron will react with copper(II) oxide to form iron oxide and copper. In this case the iron is acting as a reducing agent (*see* Chapter 5).

Metals and the Human Body
Calcium

Calcium is the most abundant metal in the human body. There will be 900–1700 g in the average (70 kg) adult and 99 per cent of this is deposited in the skeleton and the teeth. The remaining one per cent is essential for haemostasis—the concentration of calcium in platelets is five to six times the concentration in other tissues. Calcium is also influential in the metabolic reactions involved in the production of energy-rich compounds and it determines the irritability of muscle contractions. If plasma calcium is low irritability of the neuromuscular system is increased and twitching and tetany of skeletal muscles may occur, whilst increased levels of blood calcium can cause decreased muscle tonicity.

Potassium and Sodium

The average human body contains 60–100 g of sodium and 100–160 g of potassium. Sodium is the main inorganic constituent of extracellular fluid and contributes to the osmotic pressure of these fluids and so makes an important contribution to the control of body fluids. In combination with carbon (sodium bicarbonate) it forms the chief alkali reserve of the body. Sodium salts also play a part in maintaining the irritability of muscles, nerves and the heart.

Potassium is the predominant inorganic component of intracellular fluids. It is necessary for healthy growth, the transmission of nerve impulses, muscle contraction and the activation of enzymes.

The different concentration of positive sodium ions and positive potassium ions on either side of the cell membrane is possible because of the *selective permeability* of the membrane (*see* Chapter 8). This behaves as if it were impermeable to sodium, allowing potassium to enter but not to leave and not allowing sodium to enter at all.

A wide range of medicines contain sodium or potassium. They are used because many insoluble drug compounds which are not absorbed readily can be converted to soluble sodium or potassium salts which are more easily absorbed by the body. Potassium is used less often than sodium because it is less abundant and therefore more expensive. Potassium chloride (KCl) is used as a substitute for common salt (NaCl) in conditions that require a low sodium intake.

Magnesium

Most of the magnesium in the body is found in the bone tissue, of which it forms a small part. It is essential for life as it helps to maintain electrolyte balance and is involved in muscle activity. In laboratory experiments it has been found that magnesium has an anaesthetic effect on many animals and this can be counteracted with calcium. Animals become highly irritable when deprived of magnesium; convulsions, most of which prove fatal, will occur following the slightest disturbance.

Metal ions often act as enzyme activators and magnesium and manganese are frequently used. Magnesium ions (Mg^{2+}) contain two positive charges which provide a useful bridge between protein chain and substrate. (A *substrate* is a substance whose reactivity is increased by a specific enzyme.) The insoluble oxides of magnesium, magnesium oxide (MgO) and magnesium hydroxide ($Mg(OH)_2$) will be familiar to nurses as antacid powders and lotions.

Iron

Iron is essential for the formation of haemoglobin and for oxygen transport. It is present in plasma in the form of *transferrin* which carries iron to the tissues for utilization by haem and various enzymes.

Unlike some metals, iron does not accumulate in the body. The amount absorbed depends on the amount of unbound transferrin in the blood. If the concentration of transferrin in blood is saturated any excess iron will be stored temporarily in the epithelial cells of the intestine. If not used during the lifespan of the cell it will be lost when the cell is sloughed off and excreted in faeces.

Divalent ferrous sulphate ($FeSO_4$) is used in the treatment of anaemia. The trivalent compound ferric chloride ($FeCl_3$), which is readily soluble in water, is used in mouth washes. It also acts as an antidote to arsenic poisoning when added to magnesium hydroxide or sodium carbonate.

Zinc

In the body zinc is found mainly in the male testes, bone and hair. It is known to be an enzyme activator and is necessary for healthy skin.

Zinc is used in the treatment of some skin disorders. The insoluble zinc oxide (ZnO) is an ingredient of dusting powders. Zinc sulphate ($ZnSO_4$) is used in mouth washes and eye lotions.

Trace Elements

Metals such as copper, manganese and cobalt are present in the body in minute quantities only but are nevertheless essential to life. These are referred to collectively as *trace elements*.

Copper is essential for the manufacture of haemoglobin. It is transported in plasma by means of the copper protein *ceruloplasmin*, deficiency of which results in the diffusion of copper into the tissues, a condition known as Wilson's disease.

Cobalt is a constituent of vitamin B_{12} and deficiency of this metal can lead to anaemia.

Manganese is required for healthy growth and a deficiency disturbs the reproductive function of both males and females.

As already mentioned, magnesium is an important enzyme activator.

Toxicity of Metals

Some metals, for example gold and silver, have no known harmful effects. Others, such as chromium, mercury, barium and lead, are known to be harmful. Yet others, although essential 'trace elements', can be toxic in excess. Magnesium for instance, necessary for bone formation and an important enzyme activator, in excess can cause a chronic disorder of the central nervous system similar to Parkinsonism.

Occupational health nurses will be familiar with several factors which can affect toxicity, including the strength or concentration of the substance and the route of entry into the body and the ability of the substance to gain entry. This, in turn, depends on the physical state of the substance, whether a solid, and if so the size of particles, liquid or gas. Other important factors are the reactivity of the metal and the solubility of its compounds.

It is not within the scope of this book to provide a comprehensive description of the properties of toxic metals, but a brief look at some examples may serve to illustrate how reactivity and molecular structure can influence toxicity.

Chromium

Chromium is a trace element essential for glucose metabolism. In its solid state it is a hard silvery metal and is commonly used to electroplate steel to prevent corrosion. It can form six oxides. Trivalent (chromium III) and hexavalent (chromium VI) compounds are the most commonly encountered in industry. Hazards may arise from contact with chromium salts which combine with skin protein and cause skin ulceration. Improved control of mist has now virtually eliminated the effects of inhalation—ulceration and possible perforation of the nasal septum.

Trivalent compounds, if ingested, may be absorbed and will bind to organic molecules. However only 1 per cent are absorbed, unlike hexavalent compounds, 50 per cent of which are absorbed. Hexavalent compounds do not bind to organic molecules but are thought to increase the probability of lung cancer.

Mercury

This is a familiar metal, used in the manufacture of many medical and scientific instruments, not least of which is the thermometer. Mercury was known to early man who recognized its health hazards as well as its uses; consequently mines were worked primarily by convicts and slaves.

Atomic mercury has a valency of 2+ and this gives rise to mercurial compounds such as mercuric chloride ($HgCl$), a white crystalline soluble salt which is poisonous, mercuric oxide (HgO), a soluble powder which is poisonous, mercuric sulphide (HgS), an insoluble naturally occurring substance (cinnabar) used as a pigment, and mercuric fulminate ($Hg(ONC)_2$), an explosive.

Two atoms can combine to form monovalent molecules of mercury (Hg_2) which can form mercurous compounds such as mercurous chloride (Hg_2Cl_2), an insoluble powder used as a fungicide. Mercury readily forms complex ions with shared electrons and co-ordinate covalent bonds, as in organomercurial fungicidal seed dressings. These many forms of mercury cause a diversity of symptoms and before the chemistry was understood apparently conflicting reports of the signs and symptoms of poisoning appeared.

It is now known that mercury readily vaporizes at room termperature and so is easily inhaled. In its elemental form and in many of its organic and inorganic compounds, mercury is toxic to all forms of life.

Barium

Barium is a powerful muscle stimulant. Depending on the amount ingested, convulsions and death due to cardiac arrest or paralysis of the central nervous system can occur within hours, and yet 'barium meal' is used extensively as a radio-opaque medium.

The toxicity of barium depends on its absorption via the intestinal tract and this in turn depends on its solubility. The insoluble barium sulphate ($BaSO_4$) used in radiography is not absorbed, but the soluble salts of barium ($BaCO_3$, $BaCl_2$, $BaNO_2$, BaS) are rapidly absorbed and so are potentially dangerous when ingested.

Lead

Lead is an ancient metal used extensively for centuries. It is so widely deposited throughout the world that virtually no region is free of 'natural' lead pollution.

The main hazard arises out of the inhalation, and to a lesser extent the ingestion, of the dust and fumes of lead. In a solid lump it is relatively harmless but dust forms when the metal is oxidized, and this it does readily in air. Measurable amounts of fumes are produced when the lead is heated to 500 °C and over.

Lead also reacts to form organic compounds such as tetraethyl lead $(C_2H_5)_4Pb$. These are particularly hazardous and can be absorbed through the intact skin.

Poisoning by lead is a complex topic which is fully covered in almost all textbooks of occupational medicine. The following is a brief and very superficial description of its symptoms.

The classic symptoms of poisoning by inorganic lead, wrist drop, blue line on gums, anaemia, are now rarely seen in developed countries where its industrial use is controlled. In Great Britain its use is regulated by the Control of Lead at Work Regulations 1980. Early symptoms include abdominal pain, vomiting and constipation. Clinical anaemia may be detected. Encephalopathy is a serious complication which is often the presenting symptom in children.

Organic lead attacks the central nervous system and the presenting symptoms may be insomnia, irritability, tremor and mania.

Treatment of Poisoning by Metals

Poisoning by some metals is sometimes effectively treated with chelating agents. Chelation is a means of 'locking up' unwanted metal ions by surrounding them with a closed ring of compounds or radicals. *Fig.* 10.2 shows how two molecules of ETDA (ethylene diamine

tetra acetic acid) form a ring around a copper ion. *Table* 10.6 shows some of the metals that can be removed by chelation.

Haemoglobin is a naturally occurring chelating agent which 'locks up' the central iron ion.

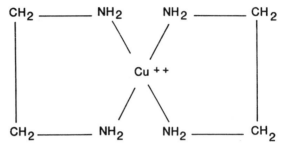

Fig. 10.2 The formation of a chelating ring around a copper ion by EDTA.

Table 10.6 Metals removed by chelating agents

Chelating agent	Metal
EDTA (ethylene diamine tetra acetic acid)	Lead
DTPA (diethylene triamine petra acetic acid)	Arsenic Chromium
BAL (British anti-Lewisite, dimercapol)	Manganese
Pencillamine	Nickel

Chelating agents can also combine with useful metals: for example, penicillamine removes calcium and iron so these will need to be replaced. Tetracycline acts as a chelating agent with calcium, magnesium, iron and aluminium and the presence of any of these in the digestive tract will inhibit the absorption of tetracycline. This will affect the timing of the administration of oral tetracycline which should not be taken immediately prior to or after the intake of food which is likely to contain such substances, but it will not affect its parenteral administration.

11

Organic chemistry

All living things, animal and vegetable, contain carbon compounds. This includes substances that are derived from living things such as the fossil fuels, coal and oil. Carbon is capable of forming a variety of structures and is the only element with this ability. It plays an important role in all living structures and the chemistry of carbon and its compounds is referred to as *organic chemistry*. Organic chemistry covers all the carbon compounds except the simple ones such as carbon monoxide, carbon dioxide, carbonates, hydrogen carbonates and carbides.

The Nature of Carbon

Carbon, with a valency of four, needs to acquire four electrons to acquire the electronic configuration of neon, a Noble gas (*see* Chapter 5)(*Fig.* 11.1). It is able to do this by pairing each of its four valence electrons with an electron from another atom. The simplest carbon compound is *methane*, in which the valence electrons of carbon are each paired

with an electron from a hydrogen atom (see *Fig.* 11.2). In combining with carbon in this way, hydrogen atoms acquire the electronic configuration of helium.

As well as forming bonds with atoms of other elements, carbon can form strong bonds with other carbon atoms. In this way stable compounds are formed which contain two or more carbon atoms (*see Fig.* 11.3).

Because carbon atoms form very stable covalent bonds they can readily form long chains, branched chains and rings (*see Fig.* 11.4).

Carbon atoms can also form double and triple bonds by sharing two or more of their valence electrons. The remaining electrons can then be paired with electrons of other elements. However, carbon cannot form *diatomic* molecules by pairing all of its electrons with another carbon atom. *Figs.* 11.5 and 11.6 show examples of double and triple bonds.

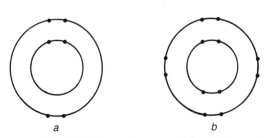

Fig. 11.1 The carbon atom (*a*) which needs to gain 4 electrons to attain the electronic configuration of neon (*b*).

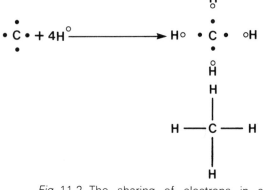

Fig. 11.2 The sharing of electrons in a molecule of methane.

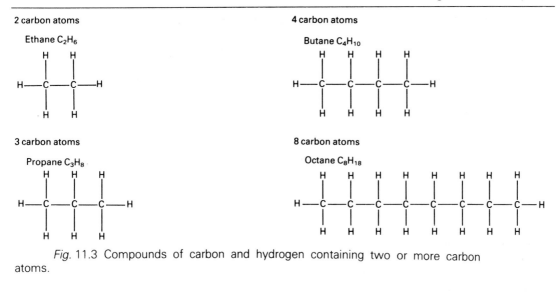

2 carbon atoms

Ethane C_2H_6

3 carbon atoms

Propane C_3H_8

4 carbon atoms

Butane C_4H_{10}

8 carbon atoms

Octane C_8H_{18}

Fig. 11.3 Compounds of carbon and hydrogen containing two or more carbon atoms.

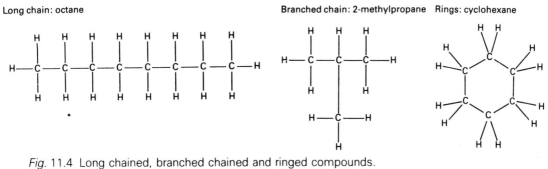

Long chain: octane

Branched chain: 2-methylpropane   Rings: cyclohexane

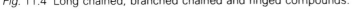

Fig. 11.4 Long chained, branched chained and ringed compounds.

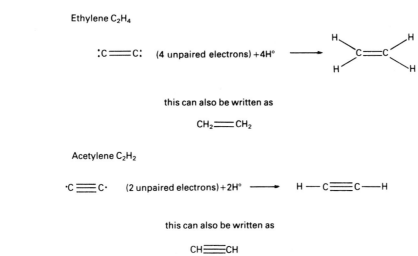

Ethylene C_2H_4

:C≡C: (4 unpaired electrons) +4H°

this can also be written as

CH_2≡≡CH_2

Acetylene C_2H_2

·C≡C·   (2 unpaired electrons) +2H°   ⟶   H — C≡C — H

this can also be written as

CH≡≡CH

Fig. 11.5 Double and triple bonds in carbon compounds.

Double bonds

Benzene

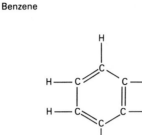

Propanone

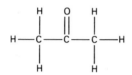

Triple bonds

Ethyne

H —— C ≡≡≡ C —— H

Fig. 11.6 Examples of organic compounds containing multiple bonds.

Properties of Organic Compounds
Melting and Boiling Points

The melting and boiling points of a substance depend upon the strength of the cohesive forces (see Chapter 8) which exist between the molecules. The stronger the force of attraction, the more heat energy is required to overcome those forces. Within any series of structurally similar molecules, the strength of the bonds increases with increasing molecular size. Generally speaking, larger molecules have higher melting and boiling points. Table 11.1 shows how boiling points increase with molecular size.

In ionic compounds, where electrostatic forces between opposing charged ions increase cohesive forces, molecular weight is still relevant (see Table 11.2).

Molecules that contain O–H bonds have higher melting points than molecules of similar structure without these bonds. This is due to hydrogen bonding (see Chapter 5).

Table 11.1 Increasing boiling points with increasing molecular weight

Compound	Molecular weight	Boiling point (°C)
Methane (CH_4)	16	−162
Ethane (C_2H_6)	30	−88
Propane (C_3H_8)	44	−42

Table 11.2 Increasing boiling points with increasing molecular weight in ionic compounds

Compound	Molecular weight	Boiling point (°C)
Sodium chloride (NaCl)	58·5	801
Lithium chloride (LiCl)	42·5	613

Solubility

A general rule is that like dissolves like. Whenever a compound dissolves, ions or molecules are separated and the spaces created are filled with molecules of the solvent. In other words, the forces between molecules are overcome and replaced by other forces. Ionic compounds which are polar (i.e. the electrons are tightly bound) can be dissolved by polar solvents such as water. Covalent compounds, which are non-polar, can be dissolved by non-polar solvents such as hexane. For example, sodium chloride will be dissolved in water, methane will be dissolved in hexane. Between these extremes many compounds will dissolve to some extent in both hexane and water. Sugar is one example; it is a covalent compound but it readily dissolves in water because glucose molecules contain O–H groups which form hydrogen bonds with water.

Reactivity

The reactivity of a compound depends on its electronic molecular structure and on the reorganization of electrons. The more loosely bound the electrons, that is the more polarizable the compound, the more easily will the bond be broken. As multiple bonds are broken more easily than single bonds compounds containing such bonds are likely to be involved in chemical reactions. For example, the single carbon–carbon bond in ethane, where the electrons have low polarity, is very strong, whereas in ethylene, which has a double carbon=carbon bond, one pair of electrons can be separated quite easily (*see Fig.* 11.7).

Ethane

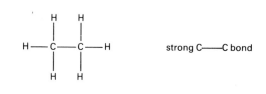

strong C——C bond

Ethylene

weaker double bond

Fig. 11.7 The relative strengths of bonds in ethane and ethylene.

Types of Chemical Change

Chemical reactions result in the building of larger molecules, or the breaking down of large molecules into smaller ones. Four different types of change can occur.

• Replacement: An atom or group of atoms is replaced by another. Benzene compounds tend to undergo this type of change, as will be shown later.

• Addition: Atoms or reagents are added to the molecule. This is a feature of compounds with multiple bonds.

• Elimination: Atoms or molecules are re-moved but not replaced—the opposite of addition.

• Rearrangement: Bonds are broken and re-formed differently, but with no loss or gain of atoms or molecules.

Organic Reaction Mechanisms

Any reaction or series of reactions will involve the breaking and making of bonds between atoms. A covalent bond between two carbon atoms, such as exists in an ethane molecule, can be broken by *homolytic* or *heterolytic* fission.

Homolytic Fission

When the bond is broken one of the two electrons in the bond goes to each carbon atom (*see Fig.* 11.8). The resulting products, each containing a single unpaired electron, are called *free radicals*. They readily undergo further reaction and so are extremely short-lived. This type of bond breaking usually occurs in the gas phase and in non-polar solvents.

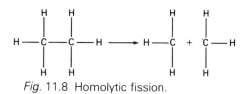

Fig. 11.8 Homolytic fission.

Heterolytic Fission

Here when the carbon bond is broken one of the carbon atoms receives both electrons (*see Fig.* 11.9). The negatively charged ion (the one which receives both electrons) is called the *carbon ion*; the positively charged ion, the *carbonium ion*. Both carbonium ions and carbon ions, like the products of homolytic fission, are free radicals and so are short-lived. They are particularly important in controlling how a particular reaction takes place, that is the sequence of steps in any reaction.

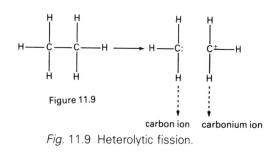

Figure 11.9

carbon ion   carbonium ion

Fig. 11.9 Heterolytic fission.

Hydrocarbons

Elements with which carbon combines to form organic compounds are usually confined to hydrogen, oxygen, nitrogen, sulphur, fluorine, chlorine, bromine, iodine and the metals. Compounds which contain carbon and hydrogen atoms only are called *hydrocarbons*.

The fossil fuels coal and oil are mixtures of hydrocarbons whilst natural gas is composed almost entirely of methane. The hydrocarbons in coal and oil need to be separated out into more useful compounds, for instance crude oil can be separated by heating to the gaseous phase and then condensing in a process called *fractional distillation* or *fractionation*. *Table* 11.3 shows some of the fractions of crude oil.

Table 11.3 Some fractions of crude oil and their uses

Number of carbon atoms	Fraction
1–4	Petroleum gases, fuel and chemical raw materials
4–12	Naphtha petrol, liquid fuel and chemical raw materials
9–16	Kerosene, jet fuel and heating oil
15–25	Diesel fuel
20–30+	Lubricating oils, waxes for candles, polishes etc.
Residue	Bitumen, road surfaces and roofing

Hydrocarbons that contain only single bonds (C–C) are called *saturated hydrocarbons*, whilst those with multiple bonds (C=C), (C≡), are called *unsaturated hydrocarbons*. Any group of compounds that fit a general formula and differ only by the number of units of that formula which a substance contains is known as a *homologous series*. Within such a series compounds will have the same chemical properties and trends in physical properties such as melting and boiling points.

Hydrocarbons fall into two broad groups, the *aromatic* and the *aliphatic* hydrocarbons.

Aliphatic Hydrocarbons
Aliphatic hydrocarbons consist of *alkanes, alkenes, alkynes* and *cycloalkanes*.

Alkanes
This series of hydrocarbons has the general formula C_nH_{2n+2}. *Table* 11.4 lists the simplest alkanes. Note that they are all derived from the same basic units (CH_2) and so are part of a homologous series.

Alkanes are saturated hydrocarbons; all

Table 11.4 Simple alkanes

Alkane	Chemical formula
Methane	CH_4
Ethane	C_2H_4
Propane	C_3H_8
Butane	C_4H_{10}
Pentane	C_5H_{12}
Hexane	C_6H_{14}
Heptane	C_7H_{16}
Octane	C_8H_{18}
Nonane	C_9H_{20}
Decane	$C_{10}H_{22}$

the bonds are single. Natural gas is largely methane CH_4 and petroleum is a mixture of alkanes up to $C_{40}H_{82}$ and other hydrocarbons. The first four alkanes in *Table* 11.4 are gases at room temperature. As the boiling point increases with chain length subsequent fractions will become liquid and then solid. Because of their single bond alkanes are unreactive; acids and alkalis have no effect on them but they burn readily with oxygen and so are often used as fuels.

Alkenes
Alkenes form another homologous series of hydrocarbons, containing a double bond. They all conform to the general molecular formula C_nH_{2n}. The simplese alkenes are ethene, propene, but-1-ene and but-2-ene (*see Fig.* 11.10).

Alkenes are obtained by cracking or splitting alkanes which have been obtained from petroleum. They can also be prepared in the laboratory. Because they contain a double bond they are unsaturated and, unlike alkanes, they are reactive. Most reactions involve addition reactions at the double carbon=carbon bond. With hydrogen, alkenes tend to form the corresponding alkane (*Fig.* 11.11a). This is the reaction which converts soft animal and vegetable oils into solid fats. With halogens, (fluorine, chlorine, bromine and iodine) they form di-chloro, di-bromo etc. compounds (*Fig.* 11.11b). Halides when added to alkenes produce haloalkanes (*Fig.* 11.11c). (A *halide* is a compound of one of the halogen elements with one other element. It is denoted by the suffix -ide, for example HBr, hydrogen bromide.)

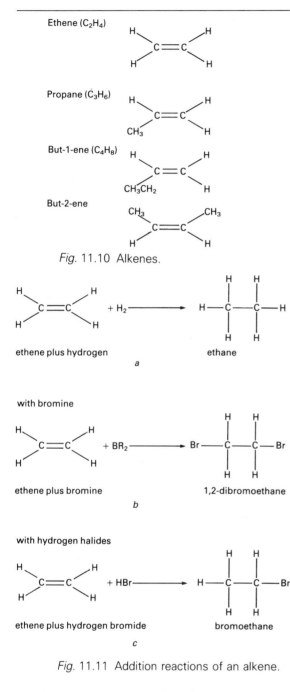

Ethene (C₂H₄)

Propane (C₃H₆)

But-1-ene (C₄H₈)

But-2-ene

Fig. 11.10 Alkenes.

ethene plus hydrogen
a

ethane

with bromine

ethene plus bromine
b

1,2-dibromoethane

with hydrogen halides

ethene plus hydrogen bromide
c

bromoethane

Fig. 11.11 Addition reactions of an alkene.

Alkenes burn in air or oxygen but because of the greater proportion of carbon atoms, they usually burn with a smokey flame.

Alkynes
All alkynes contain a triple bond and are a homologous series with the general formula C_nH_{2n-2}. The simplest alkyne is ethyne (C_2H_2).

Alkynes undergo addition reactions similar to those of alkenes. *Figure* 11.12 shows the reaction of hydrogen with ethyne with the production of ethane and hydrogen. This type of reaction usually goes straight to the alkane, without isolating the alkene stage, but it can be stopped by adding an inhibitor to stop the reaction at the second stage. This reaction takes place in the presence of a catalyst (platinum or nickel).

Ethyne can also undergo substitution reactions. This is because the hydrogen atoms in ethyne are slightly acidic. Ethyne can be distinguished from ethene by passing it into an ammonical solution of silver nitrate when silver dicarbide will be produced as a white precipitate.

Ethyne gas can be converted to benzene by passing it through a copper tube (the copper acting as a catalyst) at about 300 °C. Benzene is produced by the joining together of three molecules of ethyne (*see Fig.* 11.13).

Cycloalkanes
Cycloalkanes are saturated hydrocarbons with a ring structure. Like alkenes they have the general formula C_nH_{2n}. However, their chemical reactions closely resemble those of alkanes rather than alkenes. Cyclohexane (C_6H_{12}) is an example of a cycloalkane (*Fig.* 11.14).

Aromatic Hydrocarbons
Aromatic hydrocarbons are those that contain a ring of six carbon atoms with double and single bonds, benzene (C_6H_6) being the most important (*Fig.* 11.15).

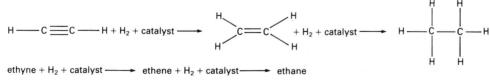

ethyne + H₂ + catalyst ⟶ ethene + H₂ + catalyst ⟶ ethane

Fig. 11.12 The reaction of ethyne with hydrogen.

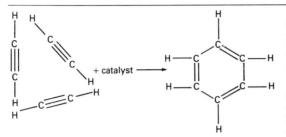

Fig. 11.13 The conversion of ethyne to benzene.

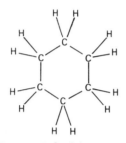

Fig. 11.14 Cyclohexane: a ring structure with single bonds.

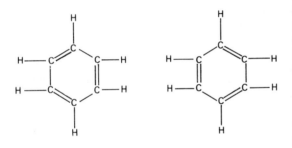

Simplified representation of a benzene ring.

Fig. 11.15 The benzene ring, showing how the single and multiple rings might be arranged.

It is usual to represent benzene in a simplified form. The two extremes represented in *Fig.* 11.15 do not actually exist. The bonds are considered to be intermediate, lying somewhere between single and double. This helps to explain why although the benzene ring contains double bonds, the ring structure is stable

and so does not readily take part in addition reactions. To do so would destroy the ring. Instead they undergo a range of substitution reactions.

Benzene is the starting point for many synthetic materials, including rubber, plastic, paints and waxes. Compounds of benzene provide a useful range of products from fungicides to explosives. Benzene is obtained from petroleum and coke. It has excellent solvent properties and in the past has been used extensively as an industrial solvent. Unfortunately its toxic properties were not recognized until long-term chronic exposure produced blood disorders, including anaemia, leucopenia, thrombocytopenia and aplastic anaemia. Voluntary agreements now exist which limit the general use of benzene to cases where it is essential, when it is used in an enclosed system. A large proportion of the benzene now produced is converted for use as intermediate products. The toxicity of benzene and its derivatives remains a problem. Polycyclic aromatic hydrocarbons, i.e. those that contain more than one ring, are now recognized as a major group of industrial carcinogens. However, now that the potential hazards have been recognized, they are more controllable.

Organic Chemicals
Classification of organic chemicals depends on the presence of certain functional groups (*see* Appendix 5).

Alcohols
Alcohols are a class of organic compounds derived from hydrocarbons by the introduction of oxygen. A primary alcohol is formed when a CH_3 group is oxidized. A secondary alcohol is formed when a CH_2 group is oxidized. Thus from ethane (CH_6) the primary alcohol ethyl alcohol is formed and from propane (C_3H_8) the secondary alcohol propylalcohol is formed. A primary alcohol will always contain a H_2COH group and a secondary alcohol will always contain a HCOH group (*Fig.* 11.16). In all alcohols the OH (hydroxyl) functional group is present.

Primary alcohol containing
the functional group H₂COH

Secondary alcohol containing
the functional group HCOH

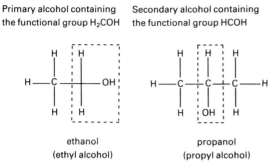

ethanol
(ethyl alcohol)

propanol
(propyl alcohol)

Fig. 11.16 Alcohols.

Ethyl alcohol is the substance commonly known as 'alcohol'. Methylated spirit is a form of ethyl alcohol to which has been added various denaturants which render it unfit for consumption. Surgical spirit, used for skin cleansing, is a solution of 70 per cent ethyl alcohol with oil of wintergreen and formaldehyde. Methyl alcohol is one of the alcohols used industrially as a solvent for lacquers and plastics and as a component of thinners and anti-freeze.

Amines

Amines are compounds in which the hydrogen atoms of ammonia (NH_3) are replaced by organic radicals. The replacement of one hydrogen atom produces a primary amine, the replacement of two hydrogen atoms produces a secondary amine, whilst replacement of all three produces a tertiary amine (*Fig.* 11.17). Unlike the alcohols, where the functional group is unchanged, in amines it is the functional group which changes. When an amine group is attached directly to a benzene ring it is called an *arylamine*.

Histamine, the substance present in body tissues which is activated by allergens to produce allergic effects, is a primary amine. Some permanent hair dyes contain primary amines which can produce allergic reaction in susceptible persons. Vitamin B_1 is a tertiary amine. The chelating agent EDTA (*see* Chapter 9) is also an amine derivative.

Some aromatic amines are known carcinogens. Beta naphthalamine causes cancer of the bladder and has been withdrawn from use in this country since 1949. In its pure state alpha naphthalamine is considered to be non-carcinogenic but it is difficult to produce in its pure form and usually contains about 4 per cent beta naphthalamine and so is considered carcinogenic to man. The difference between the two substances lies in the position of the NH_2 radical (*Fig.* 11.18). As a general rule compounds with a free position opposite the NH_2 radical are non-carcinogenic.

Benzidine was once used as a reagent for the detection of occult blood but has not

Derived from ammonia NH_3

Primary amine: replacement
of 1 hydrogen atom

Secondary amine: replacement
of 2 hydrogen atoms

Tertiary amine: replacement
of 3 hydrogen atoms

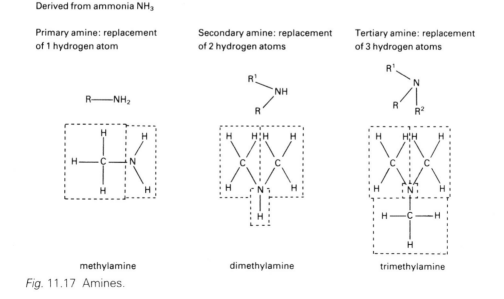

methylamine

dimethylamine

trimethylamine

Fig. 11.17 Amines.

been used for this purpose since 1962. It is still used as an intermediate in the manufacture of dyes.

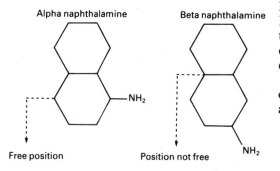

Fig. 11.18 Alpha naphthalamine and beta naphthalamine, showing the relative positions of the NH_2 radical on the benzene ring.

Esters

Esters are the product of an interaction between an organic acid and an alcohol, the hydrogen of the acid being replaced by an organic radical or group. Ethyl alcohol is the ethyl ester of acetic acid (CH_3COOH) (*Fig. 11.19*).

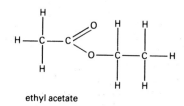

ethyl acetate

Fig. 11.19 Esters.

Esters are used as solvents and in the plastics industry as resins and plasticizers. Most organic esters are pleasant smelling solvents— methyl salicylate (oil of wintergreen) and benzyl benzoate (used for the treatment of scabies) are examples with which nurses may be familiar. Solvent esters are very powerful defatting agents.

Inorganic esters include ethyl chloride, a flammable liquid used as both a general and local anaesthetic.

Nitrates are esters of alcohols and nitric acid. Glycerol trinitrate (nitroglycerine) is the active component of dynamite and is also used as a coronary vasodilator in the treatment of angina.

Ethers

Ethers are structural isomers of alcohols (i.e. the same molecular structure but having a different arrangement and so different properties) (*Fig. 11.20*).

Ethers are used as solvents for fats and oils. Nurses will be familiar with their use as anaesthetics.

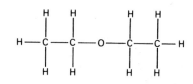

ethyl ether

Fig. 11.20 Ethers.

Ketones

Ketones are a series of compounds with a double-bonded C=O group of a general formula RR^1CO where R and R^1 are univalent hydrocarbon molecules bonded to carbon (*Fig. 11.21*).

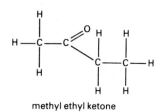

methyl ethyl ketone

Fig. 11.21 Ketones.

Ketones are highly flammable solvents which in high concentration and with prolonged exposure can be narcotic. The most important ketone is acetone which is the active ingredient of nail varnish. Ketones may be found in the urine of diabetics,

Aldehydes

Like ketones aldehydes are a series of compounds with a double-bonded C=O group but with only *one* univalent hydrocarbon radical bonded to the carbon atom (*Fig.* 11.22).

Chemically aldehydes lie between alcohols and acids. They can be reduced with hydrogen to form alcohols or oxidized with oxygen to become acids.

Formaldehyde is used for the preservation of anatomical specimens and as a fumigating agent. Paraldehyde and chloral are used to induce sleep.

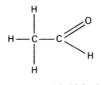

acetyl aldehyde

Fig. 11.22 Aldehydes.

Organohalogen Compounds

Often referred to as 'halogenated hydrocarbons', organohalogen compounds contain hydrocarbon molecules and one or more halogen atoms. They are non-flammable, non-combustible and non-explosive and are widely used as refrigerants and industrial solvents. The introduction of a halogen generally increases toxicity and at high temperatures they can decompose to produce free halides or halide compounds such as carbonyl halide (phosgene gas) (*Fig.* 11.23).

Organohalogen compounds are central nervous system depressants and are used as anaesthetics. Trichloroethylene, used as both an industrial solvent and an anaesthetic is probably the most widely used. Hexachlorophane is used as an antiseptic in soaps and skin cream.

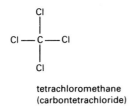

tetrachloromethane
(carbontetrachloride)

Fig. 11.23 Organohalogen compounds.

Halides

A halide is a binary compound, that is a compound of only two elements, one of which is a halogen (*Fig.* 11.24). The most important halides are formed with the metals sodium and potassium, although most other metals can form halide salts. Common salt (NaCl) is a halide of chlorine and sodium.

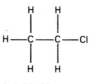

ethyl chloride
(monochloroethane)–an alkyl halide

Fig. 11.24 Halides.

Phenols

Like alcohols, phenols contain a hydroxyl (−OH) group but in phenols it is attached to a benzene ring (*Fig.* 11.25). Phenols, for example carbolic acid, have long been widely used as antiseptics and disinfectants. Today they are also used in the manufacture of phenyl formaldehyde plastics, insecticides and dye stuffs.

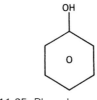

Fig. 11.25 Phenol.

Diols

Diols or glycols are compounds in which two of the hydrocarbons in an aliphatic hydrocarbon have been substituted with hydroxyl groups. They have a general formula $C_nH_{2n}(OH)$ (*Fig.* 11.26).

Diols are used as solvents and in the manufacture of plasticizers. Ethanediol (ethylene glycol) is the clear colourless viscous liquid used as an anti-freeze agent.

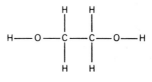

ethylene glycol (ethane diol)

Fig. 11.26 Diols (glycols).

The Chemical Industry

Before the early nineteenth century all organic compounds were derived from living or dead organisms. Then in 1828 the German chemist Friedrich Wohler, using non-organic matter, synthesized urea ($CO(NH_2)_2$) (*Fig.* 11.27). This can perhaps be seen as the beginning of the chemical industry, starting with the dye industry in the nineteenth century. Petroleum chemicals can now be converted into a wide range of products, many of which have become essential to modern living, and today man-made organic compounds far outnumber those that occur naturally. Greater understanding of chemical reactivity has increased the potential for man-made materials which now, as well as dyes, include pharmaceuticals, pesticides, detergents, paints, plastics and man-made fibres.

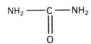

Fig. 11.27 Urea—the first organic compound to be synthesized from non-organic matter.

Many man-made and natural materials, living and non-living, exist in solid form and their strength can be attributed to their size. Many exist as giant molecules called *macromolecules*, that is molecules composed of hundreds or thousands of atoms. The strength of their chemical bonds increases with increasing size and so the stability of these giant molecules should be no surprise.

Man-made Polymers

Man-made polymers are giant molecules made up of a number of single units, *monomers*, joined together by a process known as *polymerization*. There are two types of polymerization, *addition* and *condensation*.

Addition Polymerization

This process involves the removal of a double bond and a series of addition reactions. *Fig.* 11.28 shows some familiar polymers produced in this way.

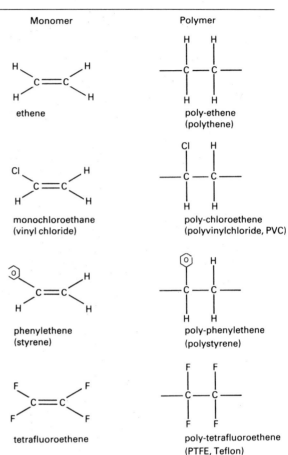

Fig. 11.28 Some familiar polymers.

Condensation Polymerization

By this reaction two molecules combine to form a larger molecule with the loss of a small molecule of water. A condensation polymer is formed following a series of reactions starting with materials that contain two reactive groups, for example HO–HO, HOOC–HOOC. Polyester (for example terylene) and nylon are produced in this way.

Cross-linking

Cross-linking between polymer chains will alter the physical properties of a polymer. It will increase relative molecular mass, affect solubility and prevent the movement of one polymer chain relative to others. It is essential to the manufacture of man-made fibres.

Natural rubber, a natural addition polymer, is not suitable for use in vehicle tyres unless treated with sulphur which hardens the rubber by forming cross-links between the chains, a process known as vulcanization.

Types of Polymers
Fibres
Fibres are polymers which are capable of being woven into textile fabrics. They are a major class of polymers.

Plastics
Plastics are substances capable of being shaped by heat or pressure. Those which soften when heated and harden again when cooled are called *thermoplastic*. Those which have hardened in the polymerization process and decompose when heated are called *thermosetting*.

Thermosetting plastics can be made more pliable by the addition of additives, called plasticizers. Polyvinylchloride (PVC) for instance is a thermosetting plastic, but the addition of plasticizers extends its usefulness.

Elastomers
Some materials, such as polythene, can be stretched but will not regain their shape when the tension is released. Cross-linking produces rigid materials which cannot be stretched at all. But a polymer with a limited amount of cross links allows a degree of movement between the molecules so that when tension is released the cross links pull the material back into its original shape. Such materials are called *elastomers*. Natural rubber is a natural elastomer, while today a large number of similar substances can be manufactured synthetically.

12

Biological molecules

The Cell

As the atom is the basic unit of all elements, so the cell is the basic unit of all living organisms. The living contents of the cell are called collectively *protoplasm*. Protoplasm, like any other material, is composed of chemical elements and so is subject to laws of chemistry and physics. The cell is, however, a highly organized collection of chemicals which are differentiated into functionally and structurally discrete parts.

Cells rely on diffusion for nutrients and oxygen and to remove waste products, so with few exceptions they are small. This helps prevent the inner part of the cell from becoming starved and hinders the build up of waste products. Some cells are flattened or elongated and this reduces the risk because all the cell contents are thus nearer the cell surface.

Cells differ from each other in shape and composition, nevertheless all cells, both animal and vegetable, possess a number of common features. Each cell is surrounded by a restraining structure—the *plasma membrane*. Inside the plasma membrane is the cytoplasm which is differentiated into different structures called *organelles*.

The Chemical Composition of the Human Body

The chemicals that make up the human body were detailed in Chapter 4. Of the total weight of an average human body, 93 per cent is made up of just three elements—oxygen 65 per cent, carbon 18 per cent and hydrogen 10 per cent. A look at the composition of the body in terms of different molecules will show that 60–80 per cent of the body is water (see *Table* 12.1).

Table 12.1 Molecular composition of the average human body

Compound	Percentage composition
Water	60–80
Protein	15–20
Lipids	3–10
Carbohydrates	1–15
Small organic molecules	0–1
Inorganic molecules (excluding water)	1

Inorganic Molecules

Table 12.1 shows the percentage of *inorganic molecules* in the body to be approximately 1 per cent. In fact inorganic substances make up about 5 per cent of the body weight but they are often chemically united with organic material, for example iron with haemoglobin, iodine with thyroxin. Many important physiological processes would be impossible without them. Enzyme activity, for instance, depends on the presence of minerals, and the osmotic pressure (*see* Chapter 8) of extracellular and intracellular fluids depends on the correct ratio of their mineral and water content. However, the exact physiological significance of some substances present is not known. Some of them are even toxic to humans when present in large enough amounts.

Water

Water is distributed unevenly throughout the body tissues, for instance dentine contains only about 10 per cent whilst 85 per cent of the brain is water. The body of an average adult male will contain about 49 litres of water and of this about 71·5 per cent will be inside the cells (intracellular) and the other 28·5 per cent outside the cells (extracellular).

The importance of water biologically lies in the fact that it is chemically neutral, it has great solvent powers and will facilitate the ionization of many substances more readily than any other medium. Many chemical and physical physiological processes would not be possible without water, for example:

- It moistens the surface of the lungs and allows gas diffusion.
- Because of its thermal conductivity and high latent heat of evaporation it plays an important role in temperature regulation. (A hand in water of 10 °C will feel cooler than in air of the same temperature because heat is conducted *from* the hand more rapidly to water than to air.)
- It provides a protective cushion for delicate structures such as the brain and spinal chord.
- It acts as a vehicle for the transport of nutrients and gases and for the removal of waste products.
- It aids the breakdown of substances such as carbohydrates by hydrolysis.
- It acts as a lubricant for moving parts such as joints, the heart and intestines.
- It is essential for the functioning of sense organs; the senses of taste and smell, for instance, are dependent on stimulation by chemical compounds in solution. Sound is conveyed to the inner ear through the fluid medium, which is largely water and it is the water in the semilunar canals which gives a sense of balance. Sight would not be possible were it not for the fluid which provides a transparent medium in the eye through which light can pass.

Organic Molecules

Many of the compounds other than water contain carbon, hydrogen and oxygen, sometimes in combination with other elements. Work on the ways in which these elements combine in the living body is a complex and continuing task, but it is possible to analyse and describe the classes of compounds present with some accuracy.

Soluble and Insoluble Fractions

The first and most crude analysis involves the separation of soluble and insoluble materials. This can easily be done by grinding a piece of tissue, such as liver or muscle, in a weak acid. The resulting suspension can then be filtered. The soluble fraction will contain almost all of the *low molecular weight substances* whilst the insoluble fraction, which will be typically whiteish or light brown, will contain the *high molecular weight* compounds.

The simplest substances which are soluble in acid are normally present in solution in the intact cell. These will be the positively charged ions—potassium, sodium, calcium, magnesium—and the negatively charged ions—chloride and phosphate. Of the organic compounds present the most important are the sugars, fatty acids, amino acids and the purine and pyrimidine bases.

Phosphates

There has already been some discussion of the physiological function and importance of the ions listed above (*see* Chapter 10). The phosphate ion, unlike other inorganic ions, combines readily with organic compounds. It therefore warrants further consideration.

Orthophosphoric acid (H_3PO_4)—a formula often written simply as Ⓟ—can readily form phosphate salts, with sodium or potassium for instance, and esters with organic alcohols. Three types of esters are possible: mono-esters, di-esters and tri-esters (*Fig.* 12.1).

Any organic compound which contains the alcohol group CH_2OH can form phosphate esters. There are, for example, sugar phosphates, amino acid phosphates, hydroxyacid phosphates, amide phosphates and nucleoside phosphates. The phosphate ester will make an otherwise inert compound very reactive, so often the first step in the metabolism (synthesis or changing) of an organic molecule will be to convert it to its phosphate ester. Combinations of phosphate groups—di- and tri-phosphate esters—are common biologically and are even more reactive than the mono-phosphate esters.

Orthophosphoric acid (H_3PO_4) can be represented by the symbol Ⓟ or diagrammatically

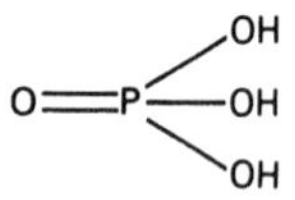

$$O = P \begin{matrix} \diagup OH \\ \text{—OH} \\ \diagdown OH \end{matrix}$$

Esters are formed with the organic alcohol CH_2OH

Mono-ester: contains 1 organic alcohol molecule

$$O = P \begin{matrix} \diagup OH \\ \text{—OH} \\ \diagdown OR \end{matrix}$$

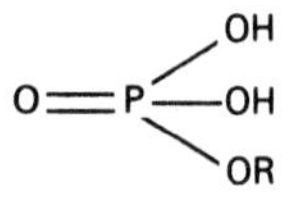

Di-ester: contains 2 organic alcohol molecules

$$O = P \begin{matrix} \diagup OH'' \\ \text{—OR'} \\ \diagdown OR \end{matrix}$$

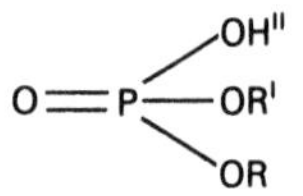

Tri-ester: contains 3 organic alcohol molecules

$$O = P \begin{matrix} \diagup OR'' \\ \text{—OR'} \\ \diagdown OR \end{matrix}$$

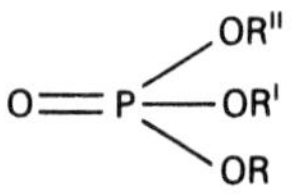

Fig. 12.1 Formation of phosphate esters (R = any alkyl group).

Organic Compounds
Fatty Acids

Fatty acids are a group of monobasic carboxylic acids composed of long hydrocarbon chains with a general formula R.COOH (R is hydrogen or a group of carbon and hydrogen atoms). They are the basic building components of many important lipids and although they are amongst the simplest substances found in the cell, they are nevertheless of great significance in the complex chemical reactions which occur in the cell. The simplest fatty acid is acetic acid (CH_3COOH).

Fatty acids are synthesized in the body with the exception of linoleic and linolenic acids. Those which the body cannot manufacture are called *essential fatty acids*. They are widely distributed in such foods as lard, peanut oil, olive oil and egg yolk.

Monosaccharides

Monosaccharides, general formula $C_nH_{2n}O_n$, are sometimes referred to as simple sugars. They are straight-chained polyhydric alcohols which are named according to the number of carbon atoms present. For example, trioses contain three carbon atoms, pentoses five and hexoses six. The molecules most relevant to human physiology are the hexoses ($C_6H_{12}O_6$). Sugars that contain an aldehyde group ($-HCO$) are aldoses, whilst those that contain a ketone group ($-CO$) are ketoses. Glucose, a hexose containing an aldehyde group, is an aldose whilst fructose is a hexose containing a ketone group and so is a ketose (*see Fig.* 12.2a). In *Fig.* 12.2a glucose and fructose are drawn as open chains in order to show the difference between them, but in reality carbohydrates do not exist as open chains. It has been suggested that they exist as ring structures, and *Fig.* 12.2b shows how the carbon 'backbone' bends to form a six-membered ring.

Blood contains about 0·1 per cent glucose, which is an essential and transportable form of energy. Ribose, found in RNA, and deoxyribose, found in DNA, are important pentoses.

Disaccharides

Two molecules of monosaccharide can combine with the loss of one molecule of water to form a disaccharide ($C_{12}H_{22}O_{11}$) (*Fig.* 12.3). Some examples of disaccharides are:
- sucrose = glucose and fructose
- maltose = glucose and glucose
- lactose = glucose and galactose.

Monosaccharides and disaccharides are sweet, crystallizable, soluble and dialysable. They are the basic constituents of carbohydrates.

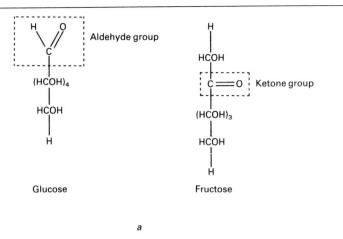

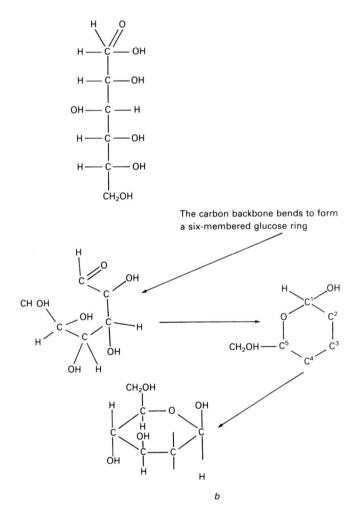

Fig. 12.2 Glucose and fructose.

$$C_6H_{12}O_6 + C_6H_{12}O_6 \rightarrow C_{12}H_{22}O_{11} + H_2O$$

glucose + fructose − sucrose + water

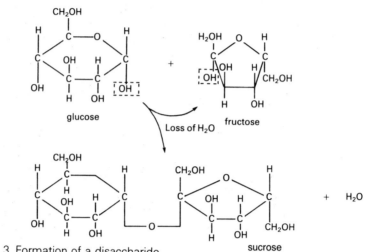

Fig. 12.3 Formation of a disaccharide.

Amino Acids

Organic acid molecules contain a carboxyl group (COOH) which confers acidic properties and facilitates combination with basic substances to form organic salts. For example, acetic acid combines with sodium hydroxide to form sodium acetate and water (*Fig.* 12.4).

A reaction in which one of the hydrogen atoms of the CH_3 group of the acetic acid is replaced with an amino group, NH_2, will produce an *amino acid* (*Fig.* 12.5).

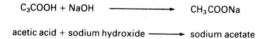

$$C_3COOH + NaOH \longrightarrow CH_3COONa$$

acetic acid + sodium hydroxide ⟶ sodium acetate

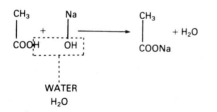

Fig. 12.4 Formation of an organic salt: combination of acetic acid and sodium hydroxide.

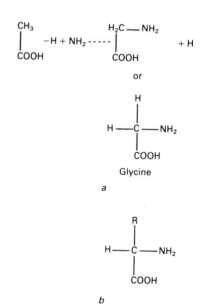

Fig. 12.5 (*a*), The formation of an amino acid (glycine) and (*b*) the general formula for amino acids. R can represent a number of groups. In glycine, the simplest amino acid, R = hydrogen.

Zwitterions

Amino acids are characterized by the presence of an acidic carboxyl group *and* an alkaline amino group. In solution both acidic and basic groups are ionized to form dipolar ions. Ions such as these, which contain both positive and negative charges, are called *zwitterions*. *Fig.* 12.6 represents the formula of an ionized amino acid.

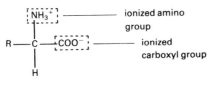

Fig. 12.6 An ionized amino acid.

Zwitterions have interesting chemical characteristics which are retained when they combine to form proteins. When an acid is added to a neutral solution of amino acid, hydrogen ions will combine with the ionized carboxyl group so conferring a net positive charge. An alkali added to a similar neutral solution will result in the hydroxyl ion removing the hydrogen from the amino acid, leaving the zwitterion with a net negative charge. The pH of the solution surrounding an amino acid will, therefore, determine whether the amino acid is neutral or whether it carries a positive or negative charge.

Essential amino acids are necessary to maintain growth and nitrogen balance. Like essential fatty acids they cannot be synthesized by the body and so must be supplied in the diet. Formation of proteins depends on the presence of all necessary amino acids simultaneously, and as they are not stored to any great extent essential amino acids must all be taken at the same time.

There are 22 amino acids. They are all similar by virtue of the presence of an amino group (NH_3) and a carboxyl group (COOH), and different in the composition of the rest of the molecule. Some amino acids belong to the *aromatic* group of compounds in which the carbon atoms are arranged to form a ring structure. The parent substance of all the aromatic substances is benzene (C_6H_6) (*see* Chapter 11).

Since molecules of amino acids are both acidic and basic they can combine with each other to form bigger and more complex molecules. Compounds formed by the union of two amino acids are called *dipeptides*. Like individual amino acids they contain a carboxyl and an amino group and so a dipeptide can unite with another amino acid to form a *tripeptide*. This union of amino acids is called *peptide linkage*.

Purines and Pyrimidines

Purines and pyrmidines are two simple related ring compounds which are the building blocks of the nucleic acids (*Fig.* 12.7).

Cytosine, uracil and thymine are examples of pyrimidines and the commonest purines are adenine and guanine. They are usually combined with the sugar ribose and one or more phosphate groups, when they are known as *neucleotides*.

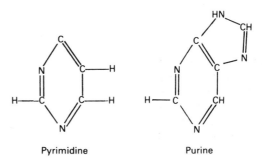

Pyrimidine   Purine

Fig. 12.7 Purines and pyrimidines.

Biological Macromolecules

In the same way that single units of hydrocarbons (monomers) can combine to form macromolecules (polymers), so single units of biomolecules can combine to form giant biological molecules—carbohydrates, lipids, proteins and nucleic acids—which form a major part of all living organisms.

Carbohydrates

Monosaccharides and disaccharides, which have already been considered, are two of the three classes of carbohydrates; the third is the *polysaccharides*.

Polysaccharides are condensation products of monosaccharides. The process whereby monosaccharides combine to form disaccharides, with the loss of a molecule of water, can be repeated indefinitely. This is the way in which polysaccharides are formed, with the loss of one water molecule for each unit of monosaccharide combined.

Within any such molecule there is scope for great variation. For instance, it is possible to alter any or all of the sugar units to produce straight chains and branched chains, which can themselves branch out, like a tree. A polysaccharide can contain 1000 units and any of these may be a different monosaccharide (for example a hexose or pentose) or a different isomer of any of them. There are, for instance, 16 known hexose isomers.

Most polysaccharides are vegetable in origin and are widely distributed as starches and cellulose. In plants they form important structural compounds, a function which in animals is fulfilled by lipids and proteins. In animals, including man, polysaccharides occur in the form of glycogen. It is found mainly in the liver and muscles and is the form in which carbohydrates are stored in man. Glycogen can be broken down into monosaccharides (glucose) by enzyme activity (or outside the body by boiling with a strong acid). In this case one molecule of water will be added for each unit of monosaccharide liberated, a process known as *hydrolysis* or *hydrolytic cleavage*.

Lipids

Fatty acids are the basic units from which lipids are formed. Their presence, together with solubility in such solvents as alcohol, ether and chloroform, is characteristic of lipids. They vary from straight-chained hydrocarbons such as fats and waxes (*see* Chapter 11) to more complex substances, such as phospholipids and steroids.

Fats

Fats are a combination of straight-chained fatty acids containing 16–18 carbon atoms and glycol. In humans, fat, like glycogen, is a means of storing energy (food). Surplus food is converted to *adipose tissue*. Fat also serves as a protective cushion for organs, such as the kidneys, and subcutaneous fat acts as an insulator.

Phospholipids

Phospholipids contain, in addition to fatty acids and glycerol, phosphoric acid and a nitrogen compound such as amino acid. Phospholipids are important structural components of the cell and nerve tissue.

Steroids

Steroids differ in both structure and function from either fats or phospholipids. They are included in the lipid group because of their solubility in organic solvents. The basic structural pattern is of 17 carbon atoms linked to form four interlocking carbon rings (*Fig.* 12.8).

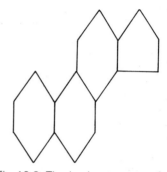

Fig. 12.8 The basic structure of a steroid.

Cholesterol is a typical steroid and is an important intermediate in the synthesis of other important steroids such as vitamin D, drugs, bile salts and hormones.

Proteins

Proteins are the group of macromolecules which are fundamental to the structure and function of *all* living things. They are formed by the linking of amino acids to form polypeptide chains, the amine group of one amino acid being joined to the carboxyl group of another in what is known as a *peptide bond*. Unlike polysaccharides, proteins are never branched, but this is about the only feature of proteins which is simple!

Proteins can differ in the total number of amino acids in the polypeptide chain, the relative numbers of each present and the way in which they are arranged. The diversity of structures possible can perhaps be more readily appreciated by considering the following examples.

A protein containing only four amino acids in which each one is used only once can yield 24 different structures. The number of possible structures when one of each of the known 22 amino acids combines is 39×10^{25}. When 600 or more amino acids combine, as they often do, then the possible permutations defy calculation. It is not surprising, therefore, that proteins are the most complex of all chemical compounds. Most of the energy of the cell is used in their synthesis and in making them work in a multitude of ways.

Proteins are generally regarded as colloids (see Chapter 9) and can behave as either acids or bases. This is a characteristic retained from the basic amino acids which gives to proteins the property responsible for the buffering action (see Chapter 9) in blood and other tissues. Most proteins will retain their biological properties only within a very narrow range of pH and temperature, and this makes it very difficult, sometimes impossible, to determine their exact structure and shape.

Simple and Conjugated Proteins
According to their composition, proteins can be divided into two classes, simple and conjugated proteins. Simple proteins contain only amino acids and have little functional significance. Conjugated proteins are composed of simple proteins united with another substance such as a pigment, nucleic acid, phosphoric acid or lipid.

Protein Structure
Structurally proteins fall into two main classes, fibrous and globular.

Fibrous proteins are, as the name implies, long fibres or sheets of polypeptide chains arranged in parallel rows. They are tough, insoluble in water and form the structural components of connective tissue. Globular proteins are polypeptide chains which are arranged in spherical or globular shapes. They are soluble in water and chemically very reactive.

Protein Function
Because of their wide variation in size and structure, proteins are capable of a wide range of functions. Some, for instance, are enzymes, some hormones, some antibodies, others, such as keratin and collagen, have a structural role.

Enzymes
Enzymes have a vital role to play because cellular activity would not be possible without them. The end product of a cellular reaction depends entirely on the materials or substrates on which the enzyme acts; the enzyme itself, like the catalyst of chemical reactions, remains unchanged. Some enzymes depend on one or more non-protein substances, co-factors, for their reactivity. This might be an organic molecule known as a co-enzyme or a metal ion or both.

Each enzyme is specific and will only react with certain groups of compounds, or in some cases with only a single compound. It is able to do this by virtue of its shape or structural configuration, rather like a lock and key.

A standardized nomenclature in which the suffix -ase is appended to the name of the substrate is a convenient way of identifying enzymes. For example the specific enzyme for urea is urease. However, enzymes which have long been recognized and whose names are familiar, such as pepsin and tripsin, will undoubtedly continue to be known by their familiar names.

Nucleic Acids
The complex organic acids DNA and RNA are made up of nucleotide units (dirobose or deoxyribose linked to purine or pyrimidine bases). DNA (deoxyribonucleic acid) is the hereditary material of most living organisms, the exception being some viruses, in which the hereditary material is RNA. The DNA molecule consists of a double helix of two polynucleotide chains which are linked by hydrogen bonds. The number of purine bases (adenine and guanine) and pyrimidine bases (cytosine and thymine) are equal and this allows the bonding between them to be very specific, which enables DNA to produce exact copies of itself during cell division, a process known as replication.

RNA (ribonucleic acid) is usually composed of a single strand of nucleotides each containing a sugar (ribose as opposed to the deoxyribose in DNA), phosphoric acid and one of four nitrogenous bases—adenine, guanine, cytosine and uracil (uracil as opposed to the thymine of DNA). It is synthesized in the nucleus by DNA and distributed throughout the cell where it directs protein synthesis.

ATP (adenosine nucleotide triphosphate) is well known as the molecule which 'stores' energy. This is made up of the purine base adenine linked to D-ribose combined with triphosphate. The release of a large amount of energy would be wasteful, most would be dissipated as heat, which could damage or destroy the cell. To avoid this glucose is broken down in a series of reactions, each of which releases a small amount of energy. Adenosine, the nucleotide formed from adenine and ribose, can be phosphorylated to yield first adenosine monophosphate (AMP), then adenosine diphosphate (ADP) and finally adenosine triphosphate (ATP). Hydrolysis of the two terminal phosphates of ATP yields 8000 calories from each and hydrolysis of the third, 3000. The essential difference between the three molecules is, therefore, that ATP and ADP are *energy-rich* and AMP is *energy-poor*. Energy-rich bonds provide a convenient method of storing the energy released by glucose oxidation. In the series of steps involved in the oxidation of CO_2, whenever a reaction yields more than 8000 calories a molecule of ATP can be synthesized from a molecule of ADP. When the cell has used 8000 calories of energy a molecule of ATP will be hydrolysed to release ADP and a phosphate.

Many different reactions can provide ATP and many different ones draw on the calories locked up. ATP is made during glucose, fatty acid and amino acid breakdown and is split in the synthesis of macromolecules, the contraction of muscles, the transmission of nerve impulses and the transport of nutrients and waste products.

Mono-, di- and triphosphate groups are all possible and the addition of any one of these groups to any substances renders the molecule biologically reactive. In accord with this general rule, nucleotides, particularly their triphosphates, are the most highly reactive of all biological molecules.

Characteristics of Life

Living organisms are made up of atoms of the same elements as inanimate objects and are subject to the same laws of chemistry and physics. This gives rise to the age-old question—what is life? The following physiological functions are ways in which living organisms differ from other objects and so constitute the characteristics of life.

- Nutrition: All living things take substances from their environment which provides energy and materials for growth.
- Growth: There will be increase in size and complexity—consider for example growth from a fertilized ovum to an adult human.
- Respiration: The way in which energy is made available to the cell. This includes the exchange of gases with the environment and the production of ATP by the cell.
- Excretion: The removal of waste products of metabolism from the body.
- Reproduction: An organism must be able to reproduce itself if it is not to become extinct.
- Sensitivity: The ability of the organism to react with its environment.
- Mobility: Movement of part or whole of the organism is the most obvious sign of sensitivity.

None of these characteristics, however, explains the essential *difference* between living and non-living things. Perhaps the question should not be 'what are living things made of?' but 'what is it that allows living things to continue to exist?'. In order to find out what elements make up living things, biochemists must destroy tissue and reduce the living body to an assortment of chemicals. But this is not to say that living cells and molecules differ in composition and structure from non-living ones.

The large molecules (macromolecules) which have been described and which make up living things are all complex and can only be synthesized in the body in accord with very precise plans (*metabolic pathways*) which involve highly specific reactions. Most of these molecules defy reproduction by the biochemist. One essential feature of a living organism is that it is a dynamic system. The molecules that make up a living system are all highly unstable and so are constantly changing, with molecules being constantly broken down and renewed.

Few molecules survive more than a few days and therefore one very important function of the living cell is its own re-creation. Being able to survive only within relatively narrow limits of temperature and pH, molecules and the living organisms of which they are a part, can adjust to environmental changes, but only minor ones.

A totally satisfactory answer to the question 'what is life?' has yet to be found. Life is a continuous and constant stimulus–response process in which the living organism must adjust to the environment or adjust the environment to itself if it is to survive. But it is only by understanding the scientific laws which govern the universe and all things in it that the environment can be adjusted and controlled.

Appendix 1 Numbers and notations

Factors and Multiples

When a whole number, called an integer, is exactly divisible by another number (that is, when nothing remains) then the first number is called a *factor* and the second is called a *multiple*. Thus, in the example 16 divided by 2, 2 is a factor of 16 and 16 is a multiple of 2.

Powers and Indices

A whole number is sometimes written followed by a superscript, for example 2^4. This is known as *index notation*. The whole number is called the *base* and the superscript is called the *index*. In the examples 2^4 and 3^3 the whole numbers 2 and 3 are bases and the superscripts 4 and 3 are indices.

The word *power* can be used instead of index so that 2^4 is 2 to the power of 4, which is another way of writing $2 \times 2 \times 2 \times 2 \, (= 16)$; 3^3 is 3 to the power of 3 which is another way of writing 27 or $3 \times 3 \times 3$.

This system can be used for any number, for instance: 10^4 (ten to the power of 4) or $10 \times 10 \times 10 \times 10$ or 10000.

Standard Form

Because of the convenience of using the method to the base 10, this method is frequently used for writing large numbers and is known as *standard form*.

The velocity (speed) of light in a vacuum, which is 300 million metres per second, can thus be more conveniently written using standard form as 3×10^8 metres per second. By following two basic rules the use of standard form also simplifies multiplication and division.

For multiplication of the same base with different powers, add the powers. For example:

$$10^3 \times 10^4 = 10^7$$

or

$$10 \times 10 \times 10 \, (1000) \times 10 \times 10 \times 10 \times 10$$
$$(10\,000)$$
$$= 10 \times 10 \times 10 \times 10 \times 10 \times 10 \times 10$$
$$(10\,000\,000)$$

For division of the same base with different powers, subtract the powers. For example:

$$10^4 \div 10^2 = 10^2$$

or

$$10 \times 10 \times 10 \times 10 \, (10\,000) \div 10 \times 10 \, (100) =$$
$$10 \times 10 \, (100)$$

The method can also be used with negative powers to denote fractions. For example:

$$10^{-1} = 1/10$$
$$10^{-2} = 1/100$$
$$10^{-3} = 1/1000$$
$$10^{-4} = 1/10\,000$$

Negative indices can also be used in place of the solidus to represent the word 'per', thus metres per second can be written as m/s or as ms^{-1}. Acceleration, which is measured in metres per second per second, can thus be written ms^{-2}.

Measurements in the universe range from the estimated size of the universe (10^{25} Mm) to the diameter of an atomic nucleus (10^{-14} m) and less. Not only is it far less cumbersome to write these numbers using powers and indices, it is also safer for they are far less likely to be written incorrectly.

Logarithms

Logarithm is another word for power or index. The word *logarithm* is used when multiplication and division are replaced by addition and subtraction of indices. Base 10 is commonly used, when the indices are called *common logarithms*. For example, $100 = 10^2$ so 2 is the logarithm of 10 and this can be expressed as:

$$\log_{10} 100 = 2 \quad (\log = \text{logarithm}).$$

Not all common logarithms are whole numbers; for instance

$$\log_{10} 2 = 0.301 \text{ or } 2 = 10^{0.3}.$$

The common logarithms of all numbers between 1 and 10 (to four significant figures) have been listed in logarithmic tables (*log tables*). Because logarithms are indices, they obey the rules of indices and this makes calculations much easier.

Log tables can be used to find the value of any number between 1 and 10 as a power of 10. For example $5·5 = 10^{0.073}$. The tables can also be used to change a power of 10 into a number value.

Appendix 2 Spectrum of electromagnetic radiations

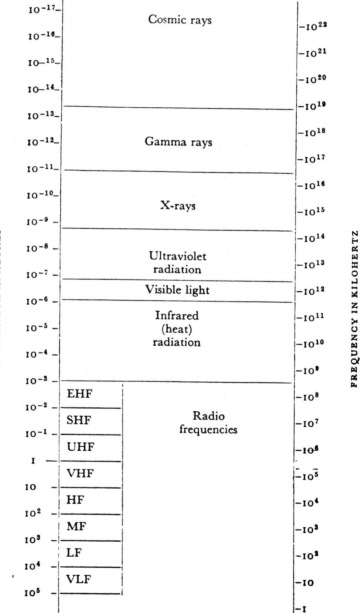

WAVE LENGTH IN METRES

FREQUENCY IN KILOHERTZ

10^{-17}	Cosmic rays
10^{-16}	
10^{-15}	
10^{-14}	
10^{-13}	
10^{-12}	Gamma rays
10^{-11}	
10^{-10}	X-rays
10^{-9}	
10^{-8}	Ultraviolet radiation
10^{-7}	
	Visible light
10^{-6}	
10^{-5}	Infrared (heat) radiation
10^{-4}	
10^{-3}	

EHF, SHF, UHF, VHF, HF, MF, LF, VLF — Radio frequencies

10^{22}, 10^{21}, 10^{20}, 10^{19}, 10^{18}, 10^{17}, 10^{16}, 10^{15}, 10^{14}, 10^{13}, 10^{12}, 10^{11}, 10^{10}, 10^{9}, 10^{8}, 10^{7}, 10^{6}, 10^{5}, 10^{4}, 10^{3}, 10^{2}, 10, 1

Appendix 3 Basic measures and SI units

Basic Measures

All measurements are based on arbitrary measures which must be permanent and reproducible if they are to be useful. Once standard units for fundamental quantities such as length, mass and time have been agreed, other quantities can be expressed as multiples of these units. It is because the choice is arbitrary that many systems have been used over the centuries.

Early units were based on readily available objects. The human body was thus the basis for such units as the cubit, the distance between the middle finger and the elbow, the hand, the width of a man's hand and still used as a measure for horses; the inch, the width of the thumb; foot, the length of a foot; and yard, the distance from the nose to the end of the middle finger. The stone (i.e. 14 lb) is a relic of the Babylonians who used stones as standard weights, whilst the grain survives from the time when Egyptians used a grain of corn as a standard measure.

Although somewhat rough and ready, all of these and many other units met the requirements of their time. Over the centuries with the development of commerce and the advance of scientific inquiry there rose a need for more accuracy and standardization. Then in 1960 the General Conference of Weights and Measures approved the universal adoption of a system called *Système International d'Unites* (abbreviated to SI units in all languages). There are seven basic SI units and from these all other measures can be derived (*Table* 1).

Table 1 Basic SI units

Basic unit	Measure of	Abbreviation
metre	length	m
kilogramme	mass	kg
second	time	s
ampere	electric current	A
kelvin	temperature	K
mole	amount of a substance	mol
candela	luminous intensity	cd

The Units Explained
Metre—the Unit of Length

The metre was originally defined as one ten millionth of the distance from the pole to the equator measured along the line of a circle passing through Dunkirk (France) and a place close to Barcelona (Spain). This distance could be remeasured at will and certainly could not be lost; but it was somewhat inconvenient and one wonders who thought this one up! Instead, two marks one metre apart were inscribed on a metal bar, the original being kept in a vault near Paris and copies being made for other countries. Questions arose concerning the accuracy of the copies and furthermore, because the dimensions of materials change with changes in temperature, it was necessary always to take measurements at a specific temperature. (The chosen temperature was the melting point of ice.) A more convenient base was therefore sought and found in the atom.

When an electron in an atom alters its position relative to its nucleus, it emits a pulse of light. This behaviour is easily reproducible and readily available and because each element emits a pulse of a wavelength peculiar to that element, it is a constant measure. Krypton was the element chosen and in 1960 the standard metre was defined as a length equal to 1 650 736·73 wavelengths of krypton light in a vacuum.

Kilogramme—the Unit of Mass

Mass, it will be remembered, is a measure that depends on the number and size of the atoms contained in an object. The element platinum has been chosen on which to base the unit of mass. The kilogramme is equal to the mass of a lump of platinum constructed to have a mass closely equal to that of 10^3 cm^3 (1000 cubic centimetres) of water at 4 °C. It is housed in a building near Paris.

Second—the Unit of Time

The unit of time has been based on the mean solar day, that is the average length of a day taken over a period of a whole year. The mean solar day could readily be divided into 24 hours, each hour into 60 minutes and each minute into 60 seconds. However, not only does this measure take rather a long time to reproduce, there are other problems. For instance, the earth's rotation is not regular and tidal action alters the rate at which the earth spins on its axis. So once again the properties of the atom have been utilized.

The velocity (speed) of light is the same for the light of all wavelengths and velocity = wavelength × frequency. The frequency will therefore be characteristic for any particular element and the time taken to complete a given number of cycles at any particular frequency will be constant. In 1967 caesium was adopted as the element on which to base the unit of time. The standard unit, the second, is defined as the time interval occupied by 9 192 631 770 cycles of this radiation.

Ampere—the Unit of Electric Current

The ampere is a measure of the current which, if flowing in two straight parallel wires of infinite length placed 1 metre apart in a vacuum, will produce on each wire a force of 10^{-7} newtons for each metre length.

Kelvin—the Unit of Temperature

The unit of thermodynamic temperature, the kelvin (K), is exactly the same as the temperature interval of one degree celsius (°C). The temperature of a substance is its degree of hotness and is measured on one of several different types of thermometer, some of which depend on the expansion of a liquid or gas, others on the expansion of a compound strip of two metals. Nurses will be familiar with the clinical thermometer which records the degree of expansion of liquid mercury. The principle underlying all thermometers is a graduated scale between two fixed points, the interval between these points being divided into equal parts or degrees.

On the celsius scale the upper fixed point is the temperature of steam from boiling water under standard atmospheric pressure (760 mmHg). The lower fixed point is the temperature of melting ice. The interval between these two is divided into 100 equal degrees, with melting ice being zero and steam point 100. This method of subdivision was suggested by the Swedish astronomer Celsius, after whom it was named, although it had previously been suggested by Linnaeus in 1745. Temperatures on the celsius scale are expressed in degrees (°C).

Another method of dividing the interval was devised by Fahrenheit. His scale did not use ice and steam as fixed points. He based it on the temperature of a mixture of salt and ice whose composition he did not specify and which he called 0° and the temperature of the human body, which he called 96°. On this scale ice melts at 32 °F and water boils at 212 °F. This scale is now all but obsolete, certainly in the world of science.

One of the difficulties associated with the accurate measurement of temperature is that various types of thermometer give different readings when used to measure the same temperature. This is because the measurements obtained depend on the properties of the substances used in the thermometer. In the mid-nineteenth century Lord Kelvin devised an absolute scale which he called the *thermo-*

dynamic scale (*see* Chapter 8). This is totally independent of any substance used in the thermometer.

Temperatures on the thermodynamic scale are not measured in degrees but in units called kelvins (K not °K). On this scale the melting point of ice is 273 K and the boiling point of water 373 K and it has been devised so that one unit kelvin is equal to one degree celsius. The temperature on the celsius scale can therefore readily be converted to units kelvin by adding 273.

Mole—the Unit of the Amount of a Substance

The amount of a substance which contains as many elementary units (atoms or molecules) as there are atoms in 0·012 kg (12 g) of carbon-12 is called a mole (mol). The number of molecules or atoms per mole is the same for all substances and this number ($6·02 \times 10^{23}$) is known as the *Avogadro constant* (N_A). The mass of an atom, called the *relative atomic mass* (RAM) is found by comparing it with the carbon-12 atom (*see* Chapter 2). Examples:

The RAM of carbon is 12
12 g of carbon contains $6·02 \times 10^{23}$ carbon atoms
1 mole = $6·02 \times 10^{23}$ carbon atoms

The RAM of sodium is 23
23 g of sodium contains $6·02 \times 10^{23}$ sodium atoms
1 mole of sodium = 23 g

The RAM of iodine is 127
Iodine exists as molecules (I_2) so the formula mass is 254
254 g of iodine contains $6·02 \times 10^{23}$ molecules
1 mole of iodine = 254 g

The RAM of hydrogen is 1 and of oxygen is 16
In water each molecule contains two hydrogen atoms and one oxygen atom so the formula mass is 18
18 g of water contains $6·02 \times 10^{23}$ molecules
1 mole of water = 18 g

Candela—the Unit of Light

Any source of light, a lamp for example, emits a continuous stream of energy. *Luminous flux* is the term applied to the amount of luminous energy emitted. The unit of luminous flux is the *lumen*. When light is emitted from any source luminous flux is radiated in all directions and in any particular direction light will be radiated in a small cone of *solid angle* (*Fig. 1*).

The *luminous intensity* is a measure of the luminous flux per unit solid angle. The candela is defined as the luminous intensity in the perpendicular direction of a surface of $1/600\,000$ m^2 of a black body at the temperature of freezing platinum under a pressure of $101\,325$ Nm^{-2}.

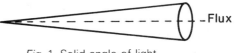

Fig. 1 Solid angle of light.

Derived Units

Derived units can be formed by combining base units, metres per second for instance. Some derived units have been assigned specific names, often in recognition of the work done by a particular person, e.g. the hertz. *Table 2* lists some of the more important derived units.

Table 2 Derived SI units

Measure of	Unit
area	metre^2
density	kilogramme/metre^3
acceleration	metre/second^2
force	newton
power	watt
momentum	newton second or kilogramme metre/second
temperature	°C
volume	metre^3
velocity	metre/second
frequency	hertz
energy	joule
pressure	newton/metre^2

When standard units are too large or too small it may be easier to express the value using powers of ten. Thus, for example, 0.0001 kg would be 10^{-4} kg and 2 750 000 m would be 2.75×10^6 m. It is, however, often more convenient to have fractional or multiple units. Those which are generally used are listed in *Table 3*.

Table 3 Fractions, multiples and prefixes

Fractions	Prefix	Symbol
$0.1 = 10^{-1}$	deci	d*
$0.01 = 10^{-2}$	centi	c*
$0.001 = 10^{-3}$	milli	m
$0.000\,001 = 10^{-6}$	micro	μ
$0.000\,000\,001 = 10^{-9}$	nano	n
$0.000\,000\,000\,001 = 10^{-12}$	pico	p
$0.000\,000\,000\,000\,001 = 10^{-15}$	femto	f
$0.000\,000\,000\,000\,000\,001 = 10^{-18}$	atto	a

Multiples	Prefix	Symbol
$10 = 10^1$	decca	da*
$100 = 10^2$	hecto	h*
$1\,000 = 10^3$	kilo	k
$1\,000\,000 = 10^6$	mega	M
$1\,000\,000\,000 = 10^9$	giga	G
$1\,000\,000\,000\,000 = 10^{12}$	tera	T

It is generally preferable to use those prefixes which change by a factor of one thousand (those which do not are marked *). An exception is the centimetre, which is often more convenient for common measurements.

The kilogramme is unusual because although it is a basic unit it is a multiple unit. When multiples or sub-multiples of the kilogramme are required they are expressed in multiples of the gramme, therefore 1/1000th of a kilogramme is 1 gramme not 1 millikilogramme.

Writing the Symbols
Units can be written out in full or the agreed symbols used. The letter 's' is never used to indicate the plural form to avoid any possible confusion with the abbreviation for second. It is not necessary to write a full stop after a symbol except at the end of a sentence. Some units commemorate the name of a person, but when written in full the names of all units, including those commemorating a person, do not have a capital letter. Symbols however do have capital letters when they commemorate a person. For example:

> newton (N)
> ampere (A)
> watt (W)
> volt (V)
> hertz (Hz)
> pascal (Pa)

When two or more symbols are combined to indicate derived units a space is left between them; for example newton metre N m. No space is left between a prefix and the symbol to which it applies; for example cm, kN, MHz, km.

The British or fps System
In this system the unit of length is the foot, of mass the pound, of time the second, and of volume the gallon. Some of the commonly used British units are given below together with conversion factors between SI and fps units (*Table 4*).

Units of length
12 inches	= 1 foot (ft)
3 feet	= 1 yard (yd)
22 yards	= 1 chain
10 chains	= 1 furlong
8 furlongs or 1760 yards	= 1 mile (mi)
6080 feet	= 1 UK nautical mile
6 feet	= 1 fathom

Units of mass
16 ounces (oz)	= 1 pound (lb)
14 pounds (lb)	= 1 stone
28 pounds	= 1 quarter
4 quarters or 112 pounds	= 1 hundredweight
20 hundredweight (cwt) or 2240 lb	= 1 ton

Units of volume
20 fluid ounces (fl. oz)	= 1 pint
2 pints (pt)	= 1 quart
4 quarts (qt)	= 1 gallon

Units of area
4840 square yards	= 1 acre
640 acres	= 1 square mile

Table 4 Conversion factors between SI and fps units

fps unit		SI unit	Reciprocal
Length	1 inch (in)	= 2·54 . 10^{-2} m	39·370 079
	1 foot (ft)	= 0·3048 m	3·280 839
	1 yard (yd)	= 0·9144 m	1·093 613
	1 fathom	= 1·8288 m	0·546 806
	1 chain	= 20·1168 m	4·970 970 × 10^{-2}
	1 furlong	= 2·01168 × 10^2 m	4·970 970 × 10^{-3}
	1 mile (mi)	= 1·609 344 × 10^3 m	6·213 712 × 10^{-4}
Area	1 in^2	= 6·4516 × 10^{-4} m^2	1·550 003 × 10^3
	1 ft^2	= 9·290 304 × 10^{-2} m^2	10·763 910
	1 yd^2	= 0·836 127 m^2	1·195 990
	1 mi^2	= 2·589 988 × 10^6 m^2	3·861 022 × 10^{-7}
	1 acre	= 4·046 856 × 10^3 m^2	2·471 054 × 10^{-4}
Volume	1 in^3	= 1·638 706 × 10^{-5} m^3	6·102 374 × 10^4
	1 ft^3	= 2·831 685 × 10^{-2} m^3	35·314 67
	1 yd^3	= 0·764 555 m^3	1·307 950
	1 fluid ounce (fl.oz)	= 2·841 306 × 10^{-5} m^3	3·519 508 × 10^4
	1 pint (pt)	= 5·682 613 × 10^{-4} m^3	1·759 754 × 10^3
	1 quart (qt)	= 1·136 523 × 10^{-3} m^3	8·798 770 × 10^2
	1 gallon (gal)	= 4·546 09 × 10^{-3} m^3	2·199 692 × 10^2
	1 bushel (bu)	= 0·036 369 m^3	27·495 944
	1 gallon USA (= 231 in^3)	= 3·785 412 × 10^{-3} m^3	2·641 721 × 10^3
Mass	1 ounce (oz)	= 2·834 952 × 10^{-2} kg	35·273 962
	1 pound (lb)	= 0·453 592 37 kg	2·204 623
	1 stone	= 6·350 293 kg	0·157 473
	1 quarter	= 12·700 586 kg	7·873 652 × 10^{-2}
	1 hundredweight (cwt)	= 50·802 345 kg	1·968 413 × 10^{-2}
	1 ton	= 1·016 047 × 10^3 kg	9·842 065 × 10^{-4}
Density	1 lb ft^{-3}	= 16·018 463 kg m^{-3}	6·242 796 × 10^{-2}
Speed	1 in s^{-1}	= 2·54 × 10^{-2} m s^{-1}	39·370 079
	1 ft s^{-1}	= 0·3048 m s^{-1}	3·280 839
	1 mi h^{-1}	= 0·447 04 m s^{-1}	2·236 936
Force	1 poundal (pdl)	= 0·138 255 N	7·233 011
	1 lbf (i.e. the wt of 1 lb mass)	= 4·448 222 N	0·224 809
Pressure	1 lbf in^{-2} (p.s.i.)	= 6·894 757 × 10^3 Pa	1·450 377 × 10^{-4}
Energy	1 ft pdl	= 4·214 011 × 10^{-2} J	23·730 360
	1 ft lbf	= 1·355 817 J	0·737 562
	1 Btu	= 1·055 06 × 10^3 J	9·478 134 × 10^{-4}
	1 therm	= 1·055 06 × 10^8 J	9·478 134 × 10^{-9}
Power	1 horse power (hp)	= 7·457 00 × 10^2 W	1·341 022 × 10^{-3}
Standard atmosphere	14·695 916 lbf in^{-2}	= 1·013 25 × 10^5 Pa	

Appendix 4 Some measures explained

Movement

Speed (s)

Speed is defined as the distance moved per second. To measure the average speed the distance travelled is divided by the time taken:

$$\text{average speed} = \frac{\text{distance moved (in metres)}}{\text{time taken (in seconds)}}$$

The derived SI unit for speed is metres per second. This can be written m/s or m s^{-1}.

Speed is a *scalar* quantity as it has only magnitude (size).

Velocity (v)

Velocity is a measurement of speed *and* direction. To measure velocity the distance moved in a particular direction is divided by the time taken:

$$\text{velocity } (v) = \frac{\text{distance moved in a particular direction (in metres)}}{\text{time taken (in seconds)}}$$

Velocity is calculated in m s^{-1} in a particular direction.

Fig. 1 shows graphs of velocity (distance moved in a particular direction against time) and illustrates how the shape of the graph varies depending upon whether velocity is uniform, increasing or decreasing.

A curve rather than a straight line on a graph represents an object whose velocity varies at different times. Velocity can change in either magnitude or direction and the direction of a force can cause an object to increase or decrease speed, to stop or veer to either side.

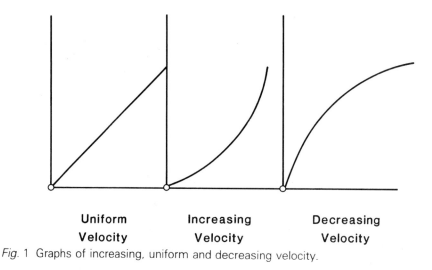

Uniform	Increasing	Decreasing
Velocity	Velocity	Velocity

Fig. 1 Graphs of increasing, uniform and decreasing velocity.

A measurement which has magnitude (size) as well as direction is called a *vector*. The voltage produced by the beating heart, which gives rise to the electrocardiogram, moves in a general direction from the centre of the chest to the left. This voltage is a vector quantity because it has both magnitude and direction.

Acceleration (a)

Acceleration is a measure of how much the speed of a moving object has increased in a given time. In other words it is a change in velocity per second.

$$\text{acceleration} = \frac{\text{change in velocity}}{\text{time taken for change to occur}}$$

If an object is at rest and after one second it is travelling at a speed of 1 m s^{-1}, then it has accelerated by 1 metre per second in one second (1 m s^{-2})—m s^{-2} means metres per second per second. Slowing down is referred to as *retardation* or *negative acceleration*. *Fig.* 2 shows the shapes of uniform and non-uniform acceleration.

Momentum

Momentum is the product of mass multiplied by velocity, so can be expressed mathematically as:

$$\text{momentum} = \text{mass} \times \text{velocity} \ (mv)$$

If the velocity of an object increases then its momentum will increase. Because it depends on velocity, momentum is a vector quantity.

Some Measures Relating to Size
Mass

This is a measure which depends on the number and size of the atoms contained in an object.

Density

The density of a substance is defined as its mass per unit volume:

$$\text{density} = \frac{\text{mass (in kilogrammes)}}{\text{volume (in cubic metres)}}$$

The SI unit of density is therefore the kilogramme per cubic metre—kg/m^3 or kg m^{-3}. The relative density of a substance is the ratio of any volume of that substance to the mass of an equal volume of water:

$$\text{relative density} = \frac{\text{mass of any volume of a substance}}{\text{mass of an equal volume of water}}$$

Measuring Work Done and Energy
Work Done

Work done has been defined in terms of force and the distance moved in the direction of the force, therefore:

$$\text{work done} = \text{force} \times \text{distance moved in the direction of the force}$$

Force is measured in newtons (N) and distance in metres (m), so the derived SI unit

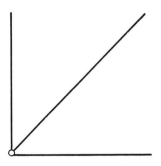

Uniform acceleration

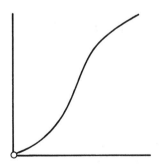

Non–Uniform acceleration

Fig. 2 Uniform and non-uniform acceleration.

of work is the newton metre (N m). The amount of work done when a force of 1 N moves through 1 m in the direction of the force is 1 N m. The newton metre has been given a specific name, the joule (J).

Pressure

Pressure is a quality which depends on force and area and can be calculated using the formula:

$$\text{pressure} = \frac{\text{force (N)}}{\text{area (m}^2)}$$

The SI unit of pressure is the newton per square metre, N/m^2 or $N\,m^{-2}$. This derived SI unit is called the pascal (Pa), although other units are sometimes used.

Atmospheric pressure is expressed in millimetres of mercury (mmHg). The average barometric pressure at sea level is 760 mmHg and this is known as *standard atmospheric pressure* or *one atmosphere*.

For meterological purposes the unit of pressure used is *the bar*. This is defined as a pressure of 10^5 newtons per square metre, $10^5\,N/m^2$ or $10^5\,N\,m^{-2}$.

The millibar, which is one thousandth of a bar, is a commonly used sub-unit:

$$1\text{ millibar} = 10^5/10^3 = 100\,N\,m^{-2}$$

Thus standard atmospheric pressure is:

760 mmHg
or 1 atmosphere
or 101 400 N m^{-2} (Pa)
or 1.014 bar
or 1014 mbar

Standard Temperature and Pressure (stp)

Because densities of gases vary to such a great extent with changes in temperature and pressure it is necessary always to record temperature and pressure in the measurements of the density or volume of any gas. For such calculations standard temperature is 0 °C and standard pressure is 760 mmHg.

Energy

Energy, which has been defined as the capacity to do work, is also measured in joules (J).

Heat Energy

Heat is energy which is transferred from one place to another because of a temperature difference. Since heat is a form of energy, this too is measured in joules (J).

The *heat capacity* of any body is the heat required to raise its temperature by 1 kelvin (1 K). The SI unit of heat capacity is therefore the joule per kelvin (J/K or $J\,K^{-1}$).

Latent or 'hidden' *heat* is the heat required to change the physical state of a substance. The specific latent heat of vaporization is the amount of heat required to change a unit mass of a substance from its liquid to its vapour state without change of temperature and is measured in joules per kilogramme (J/kg). As substances absorb heat when they melt, so they give out heat on solidifying. This is known as the 'latent heat of fusion' and is measured in the same units, J/kg. Because of the large numbers involved, sub-units, kilojoules per kilogramme or megajoules per kilogramme, are frequently used (KJ = 1000 J, MJ = 1 000 000 J).

Calorimetry

Calorimetry is the science of heat measurement. The calorie is the unit of the quantity of heat and is the amount of heat required to raise the temperature of 1 g of water through 1 °C. The International Table Calorie is defined as 4.1868 J. The kilogramme calorie, kcal or Calorie (capital C) is equal to 1000 calories and is the unit used when quoting the energy value of foods.

Waves
Wavelength

Wavelength is the distance between two successive particles which are at exactly the same point in their paths at the same time and are moving in the same direction. Wavelength is measured in metres.

Frequency

The number of complete oscillations made in one second is called the frequency and is measured in hertz (Hz), 1 Hz being one cycle per second. In one second therefore a wave moves forwards a distance of one wavelength (λ) × frequency (f). It will be remembered that:

$$\frac{\text{distance moved in a particular direction}}{\text{time taken}} = \text{velocity}$$

therefore

$$\text{frequency} \times \text{wavelength} = \text{velocity}$$

Given any two of these properties it is possible to calculate the third. For example, a wave of frequency 3 Hz and wavelength 0·8 m would have a velocity of:

$$3 \text{ Hz} \times 0\cdot8 \text{ m} = 2\cdot4 \text{ m Hz} = 2\cdot4 \text{ metres per second (m s}^{-1})$$

Sound Waves
Sound waves manifest themselves as pressure disturbances. Pressure is measured in pascals (Pa) and so this is also the SI unit used to measure sound.

Pressure
Sir Isaac Newton investigated the effects of pressure changes on the velocity of sound in air and other gases and showed theoretically that the velocity of sound is proportional to pressure.

Density
Boyle's Law states that if the pressure of a fixed mass of gas is doubled then its volume will be halved, hence the density will be doubled. At a constant temperature therefore density will remain constant regardless of any changes in pressure, thus pressure changes will not affect the velocity of sound in air.

Temperature
Change in temperature can bring about change in density without altering pressure. Therefore when the temperature increases at constant pressure air will expand and become less dense (Charles' Law). The ratio pressure/density will increase and so the velocity of sound will increase with increased temperature.

Pitch
Pitch depends on the frequency of sound vibrations. High frequency waves will produce high-pitched sound, whilst low frequency waves will produce low-pitched sounds. Generally speaking high-pitched sounds have short wavelengths and vice versa.

Intensity
Intensity is related to the quality of a sound and is a measure of the energy being emitted from the sound source. Sound energy is measured in watts (W), the derived SI unit of power equal to 1 joule per second.

Measuring Sound Levels
The sound pressures audible to the human ear range from 200 Pa to 0·000 02 Pa. Because of the inconvenience of quoting such a vast range of pressures in arithmetic units the logarithmic *decibel scale* is used. A decibel is one tenth of a bel. A *bel* is a unit which compares levels of power. The two power levels P_1 and P_2 are said to differ by n decibels when

$$n = 10 \log_{10} (P2/P1)$$

P_2 is the intensity of the sound being measured and P_1 is a chosen reference level, often the lowest audible note of the same frequency. A more detailed explanation of the decibel scale will be found in Harris (1984).

Radioactivity
Radioactivity is measured in terms of the activity of the source, the absorbed dose and the dose equivalent.

Activity of a Source
The SI unit of a radioactive source is the becquerel (Bq) which is equal to 1 nuclear disintegration per second. It can be used to measure airborne concentration, surface contamination and the specific activity of a radionuclide. The curie (Ci) is also still used. A curie is defined as the quantity of a radioactive isotope which decays at a rate of $3\cdot7 \times 10^{10}$ disintegrations per seconds. 1 Bq is equal to $2\cdot7 \times 10^{-11}$ Ci

Absorbed Dose
The SI unit of absorbed dose is the gray (Gy), named after the British radiobiologist L. H. Gray. 1 Gy of ionizing radiation is equal to the energy in joules absorbed by 1 kg of irradiated material. The old unit, which is still used, is the rad (radiation absorbed dose). 1 Gy is equal to 100 rad.

Dose Equivalent

The roentgen (R) is the unit of exposure incident on a measured surface. $1 \text{ R} = 2 \cdot 58 \times 10^{-4}$ coulomb per kilogramme. (Coulomb is the SI unit of electrical charge, *see* below.) The roentgen equivalent man (rem) is the unit dose of radiation which gives the same biological effect as that due to 1 R of X-rays. The SI unit of dose equivalent is the sievert (Sv). 1 Sv is equal to 100 rem.

Measurement of Electric Current

The strength of the flow of water in a river can be measured in terms of litres of water flowing past a given point in a river over a given period of time. Similarly the size of an electric current is a measure of the rate of flow of an electric charge past a given point in a circuit or through a conductor.

The strength of an electric current is measured in amperes (symbol A), frequently referred to as 'amps'. The ampere is a measure of a current which, if flowing in two straight parallel wires of infinite length placed one metre apart in a vacuum, will produce on each wire a force of 2×10^{-7} newtons per metre.

The quantity of an electric charge is measured in coulombs (symbol c). A coulomb is the quantity of electricity which passes any point in a circuit in one second when a steady current of 1 ampere is flowing.

Potential Difference

Potential electrical differences are measured in volts. The *potential difference* between two points is defined as the work done in joules: 1 volt represents 1 joule of work done per coulomb of electricity passing between two points of potential difference.

The total work done in joules per coulomb of electricity conveyed in a circuit is the *electromotive force* (symbol e.m.f.).

Electrical Power

The watt is the unit of power equal to 1 joule per second. The *power* in watts is given by the product of the *current* in amperes (A) and the *potential difference* in volts. One watt represents the energy expended per second by an unvarying electric current of 1 ampere flowing through a conductor the ends of which are maintained at a potential difference of 1 volt.

Reference

Harris, C. J. (ed.) *Occupational Health Nursing Practice*. Bristol, Wright, 1984, Ch. 13, Appendix 1.

Appendix 5 Facts and figures

Factual information is often given in numerical form. Data, whether gathered by observation or experiment, needs to be classified and presented in such a way that maximum information is conveyed in minimum time. Consider the following example: the ages of 30 people employed in one department could be displayed as

60	25	32	50	29	18	44	36	16	22
54	64	22	38	28	18	22	32	26	31
28	31	22	19	24	26	31	29	42	28

Here, although there are only 30 figures to consider it is difficult to learn very much about them without lengthy scrutiny. By looking carefully it can be seen that the oldest employee is 64 and the youngest 16. It is clear that the data need to be arranged so that the main features are more readily recognizable.

Classification of Data
The first step is to arrange the figures in order from youngest to oldest:

16	18	18	19	22	22	22	22	24	25
26	26	28	28	28	29	29	31	31	31
32	32	36	38	42	44	50	54	60	64

Data arranged in this way is more useable. One can, for instance, calculate averages.

Averages
Average in mathematics has more than one meaning. There are four types of average: the mid-range and mode, which are seldom used, and the median and mean.

Mid-range is the number half way between the highest and lowest. In the example given the highest number is 64 and the lowest 16, so the mid-range will be:

$$\frac{64 + 16}{2} = 40$$

Mode is the most frequently occurring number which, in our example, is 22.

In data arranged in order the *median* is the middle number of an odd number of observations and half-way between the two middle numbers in the case of an even number of observations. In the example there is an even number, so the median lies half way between 28 and 29.

$$\frac{28 + 29}{2} = 28 \cdot 5$$

The *mean* is also sometimes called the *arithmetic mean*. It is the most commonly used measure and is simply the sum of the observations divided by the number of observations. Thus

$$\frac{947}{30} = 31 \cdot 5$$

Pictorial Presentation of Data
Once data has been classified it is easier to identify important characteristics. However, a further improvement can be made by present-

ing the data in such a way that the information can be seen and understood more easily and more quickly. Some common ways of presenting data include histograms, pie charts, pictograms and graphs. In each case it will be necessary to divide the information into *class intervals* and to define *class boundaries*. The number of classes chosen must be realistic and as simple as possible. In the example previously quoted, the classes might be: under 20, 21–30, 31–40, 41–50, 51–60, over 60. It will then be possible to determine the *frequency*, that is the number of instances in each class or group, in our example the number of employees in each age group.

Histogram

A histogram presents data in bars and the area of the bar represents the frequency. (A *bar chart* is similar but here it is the height of the bar which represents the frequency) (*see* Fig. 1).

Pie Charts

Pie charts are based on sectors of a circle, with each sector proportional in area to the frequencies. For example, in a small cottage hospital there are 100 patients. Of these there are 25 in the geriatric ward, 30 in the medical ward, 20 in the surgical ward, 15 in the paediatric ward and 10 in the maternity ward (*Fig. 2*).

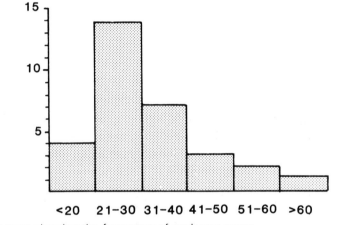

Fig. 1 Histogram showing the frequency of each age group.

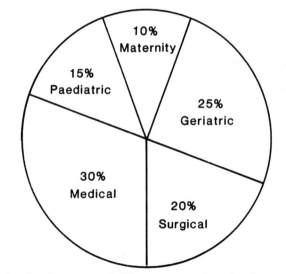

Fig. 2 Pie chart showing frequency of different categories of patient.

Pictogram

A pictogram represents data in a series of small pictures, each of which represents a given number of observations. For example, in the hospital of the last example the given symbol could represent five patients (*Fig.* 3).

Graphs

A graph is a convenient way of presenting data, to show the relationship between two quantities that vary. Whenever relationships can be put into pairs it is possible to plot these on a graph. For example, when considering the properties of a gas, the relationship between volume and pressure (Boyle's Law) or between volume and temperature (Charles' Law) or between pressure and temperature (Pressure Law) can all be shown on a graph. One example of a graph with which all nurses will be familiar is the temperature chart. This shows the relationship between temperature and time and from this it is possible to see at a glance any fluctuations in temperature as well as the temperature at any given time.

Any graph has two axes, the horizontal or X axis and the vertical or Y axis. The X and

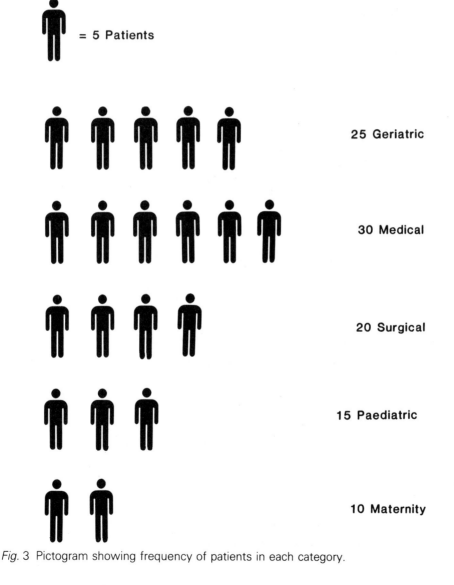

= 5 Patients

25 Geriatric

30 Medical

20 Surgical

15 Paediatric

10 Maternity

Fig. 3 Pictogram showing frequency of patients in each category.

Y axes are known as the *rectangular Cartesian axes* after the French mathematician and philosopher Rene Descartes (1595–1650). The point at which these two axes intersect is called the *origin* (0). The horizontal axis (X) is usually used for the independent variable and the line 0X is called the *abscissa*. The vertical axis (Y) is used for the dependent variable and the line 0Y is called the *ordinate* (*Fig.* 4).

On the temperature chart time represents the independent variable whilst temperature is the dependent variable, that is, it depends on time. In other instances the temperature may be the independent variable, for example, in a graph of temperature against the rate of a chemical reaction (*Fig.* 5).

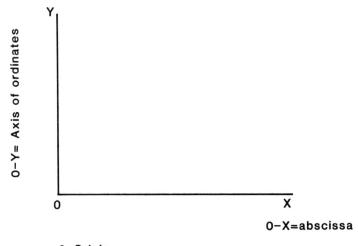

Fig. 4 The rectangular Cartesian axes of a graph.

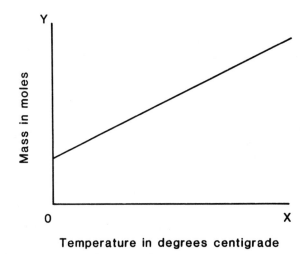

Fig. 5 Graph of temperature against rate of chemical reaction.

The Curve of the Graph

The *curve* of the graph is an expression used to describe the shape of the line drawn between the points plotted on a graph. It is called a curve even when it is a straight line. A curve indicates a direct relationship between two values: for example, a graph of distance travelled against time taken (speed) or a graph of increase or decrease in speed over time (acceleration) (*Fig.* 6).

A graph which has a regular curve can be extended or *extrapolated* to give calculated values which have not been obtained by experiment or observation.

Negative Axes

Any given quantity can be either positive or negative. The axes of the graph can be extended beyond the point of intersection (0), when negative measures will appear to the left of the horizontal axis and downward along the vertical axis (*Fig.* 7).

More Definitions
Ratio

The ratio gives a comparison between two quantities and indicates how much greater one

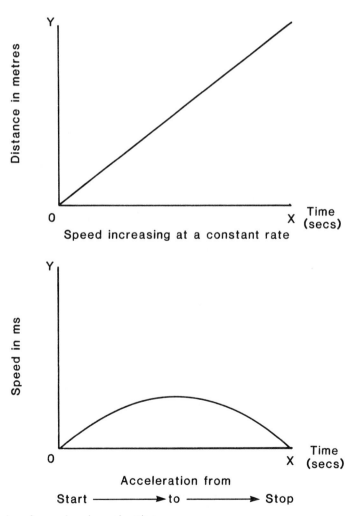

Fig. 6 Graphs of speed and acceleration.

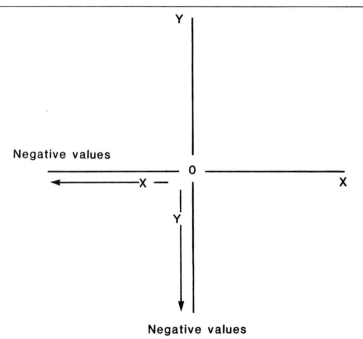

Fig. 7 Graph showing negative values.

is than the other. The two quantities must always be in the same units, for example in a molecule of water the ratio of hydrogen atoms to oxygen atoms is 2 to 1 or 2:1.

Proportion
Two quantities are in *direct proportion* when an increase (or decrease) in one is accompanied by an equal increase (or decrease) in the other. Both will be doubled, halved etc. When an increase in one quantity produces a proportionate decrease in the other (or vice versa), then the two quantities are said to be in *inverse proportion*. When one is halved the other will be doubled etc.

Probability
A number can be assigned to the likelihood of

a particular event occurring and that number is called the *probability*. A certainty has a probability of 1 and an impossibility a probability of 0, so probability is expressed as a value lying between 0 and 1. For instance, a die has six sides numbered 1–6. When a die is tossed the probability of any one number, say 4, turning up will be 1/6 or 1 in 6. (A more detailed explanation of probability will be found in Harris, 1984).

Reference
Harris, C. J. (ed.) *Occupational Health Nursing Practice*. Bristol, Wright, 1984, Ch. 2.

Appendix 6 Chemical symbols formulae

Chemical symbols are used to identify elements. Usually the initial letter or first two letters of its name are used, for instance:

Carbon C
Nitrogen N
Chlorine Cl

Sometimes the first letter (or first two letters) of the Latin name of an element are used, for instance:

Iron (Latin *ferrum*) Fe
Copper (Latin *cuprum*) Cu
Gold (Latin *aurum*) Au

Table 1 lists all the elements together with their symbols.

When two or more atoms of the same element combine to form molecules of that element, this is represented by the chemical symbol followed by a subscript to indicate the number of atoms in combination, for instance: $O_2 = 2$ atoms of oxygen in combination (atmospheric oxygen); $O_3 = 3$ atoms of oxygen in combination (ozone).

Molecules of combinations of two or more atoms of different elements (compounds) can be represented in the same way, for instance: NaCl = 1 sodium atom + 1 chlorine atom (sodium chloride); H_2O = 2 hydrogen atoms + 1 oxygen atom (water).

Chemical Formulae

The chemical symbols of elements, molecules and compounds presented in this way indicate the relative proportions of the different elements which they contain, in other words they give a *formula*. A whole number which precedes a formula indicates the number of parts contained in the substance, for instance 2HCl indicates two molecules of hydrogen chloride. A number that follows a bracket multiplies everything in that bracket, for instance $(NH_4)_2SO_4 = 2$ molecules of NH_4 and 1 molecule of SO_4.

Chemical formulae are used to indicate the composition of a substance: they are not a shorthand description of that substance. For instance, all that can be learned from the formula for sugar, $C_{12}H_{22}O_{11}$, is that it consists of 12 carbon atoms, 22 hydrogen atoms and 11 oxygen atoms.

Formulae can also be drawn as structures, which give more information about how the atoms are linked together (*Fig.* 1).

Isomers

Two quite different compounds may have the same overall formula. These are known as *isomers*. But they will exhibit different properties because of the different arrangement of atoms in the molecule. For example, ammonium cyanate and urea have the same basic formula—N_2H_4CO. In such cases the formula can be written in extended form and this will show something of the internal structure of the molecule.

Ammonium cyanate NH_4CNO
Urea $CO(NH_2)_2$

Atomic Numbers (Z)

The number of protons in an atom is known as

121

Table 1 Elements with their atomic number and symbol

Atomic number (Z)	Symbol	Name	Atomic number (Z)	Symbol	Name
1	H	Hydrogen	54	Xe	Xenon
2	He	Helium	55	Cs	Caesium
3	Li	Lithium	56	Ba	Barium
4	Be	Beryllium	57	La	Lanthanum
5	B	Boron	58	Ce	Cerium
6	C	Carbon	59	Pr	Praseodymium
7	N	Nitrogen	60	Nd	Neodymium
8	O	Oxygen	61	Pm	Promethium
9	F	Fluorine	62	Sm	Samarium
10	Ne	Neon	63	Eu	Europium
11	Na	Sodium	64	Gd	Gadolinium
12	Mg	Magnesium	65	Tb	Terbium
13	Al	Aluminium	66	Dy	Dysprosium
14	Si	Silicon	67	Ho	Holmium
15	P	Phosphorus	68	Er	Erbium
16	S	Sulphur	69	Tm	Thulium
17	Cl	Chlorine	70	Yb	Ytterbium
18	A	Argon	71	Lu	Lutetium
19	K	Potassium	72	Hf	Hafnium
20	Ca	Calcium	73	Ta	Tantalum
21	Sc	Scandium	74	W	Tungsten
22	Ti	Titanium	75	Re	Rhenium
23	V	Vanadium	76	Os	Osmium
24	Cr	Chromium	77	Ir	Iridium
25	Mn	Manganese	78	Pt	Platinum
26	Fe	Iron	79	Au	Gold
27	Co	Cobalt	80	Hg	Mercury
28	Ni	Nickel	81	Tl	Thallium
29	Cu	Copper	82	Pb	Lead
30	Zn	Zinc	83	Bi	Bismuth
31	Ga	Gallium	84	Po	Polonium
32	Ge	Germanium	85	At	*Astatine*
33	As	Arsenic	86	Rn	Radon
34	Se	Selenium	87	Fr	*Francium*
35	Br	Bromine	88	Ra	Radium
36	Kr	Krypton	89	Ac	Actinium
37	Rb	Rubidium	90	Th	Thorium
38	Sr	Strontium	91	Pa	Protactinium
39	Y	Yttrium	92	U	Uranium
40	Zr	Zircinium	93	Np	*Neptunium*
41	Nb	Niobium	94	Pu	*Plutonium*
42	Mo	Molybdenum	95	Am	*Americium*
43	Tc	*Technetium*	96	Cm	*Curium*
44	Ru	Ruthenium	97	Bk	*Berkelium*
45	Rh	Rhodium	98	Cf	*Californium*
46	Pd	Palladium	99	E	*Einsteinium*
47	Ag	Silver	100	Fm	*Fermium*
48	Cd	Cadmium	101	Mv	*Mendelevium*
49	In	Indium	102	No	*Nobelium*
50	Sn	Tin	103	Lw	*Lawrencium*
51	Sb	Antimony	104	Ku	*Kurchatovium*
52	Te	Tellerium	105	Ha	*Hahnium*
53	I	Iodine			

The elements printed in italic do not occur naturally, but have been produced artificially.

Water H_2O

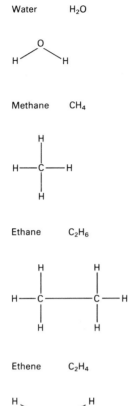

Methane CH_4

Ethane C_2H_6

Ethene C_2H_4

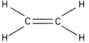

Fig. 1 Representations of water, methane, ethane and ethene.

the atomic number and is represented by a subscript which precedes the chemical symbol, for instance

Carbon $_6C$
Hydrogen $_1H$

Mass Numbers (A)
The total number of nucleons (protons and neutrons) in an atom is known as the *mass number* and is represented by a superscript which precedes the chemical symbol, for instance

Hydrogen ^1H
Carbon ^{12}C

Isotopes (*see* Chapter 4)
By indicating the atomic number and the mass number different isotopes of a particular atom can be identified, for instance:

The three isotopes of hydrogen $_1^1H$ $_1^2H$ $_1^3H$

The three isotopes of carbon $_6^{12}C$ $_6^{13}C$ $_6^{14}C$

As the atomic number defines the specific element, it is not normally necessary to specify both the atomic number and chemical symbol. It is usual to omit the atomic number subscript and so the isotopes of carbon would normally be written:

$$^{12}C \quad ^{13}C \quad ^{14}C$$

These isotopes are referred to in speech as carbon (or C-12, C-13 and C-14).

Ions
Ions are represented by the chemical symbol followed by a superscript indicating the charge, for instance:

Lithium (a positive ion) Li^+
Calcium (a double positive ion) Ca^{2+}
Fluoride (a negative ion) F^-
Sulphide (a double negative ion) S^{2-}

Elements of Groups I, II and III form positive ions and retain the name of the element (lithium, beryllium etc.), whilst elements of Groups VI and VII form negative ions and the name of the element changes to end in 'ide' (oxide, fluoride, chloride etc.).
In forming ionic compounds, the number of positive charges will equal the number of negative charges. Sodium chloride, for instance, contains Na^+ ions and Cl^- ions, so the ratio of Na to Cl will be $1:1$ (formula NaCl). However, sodium sulphate contains Na^+ ions and SO_4^{-2} ions, so the ratio of Na to SO_4 will be $2:1$ (formula Na_2SO_4).

Chemical Equations
Atoms can neither be created nor destroyed, so when a chemical reaction occurs, atoms which are present in the original substance will merely be reshuffled. It must, therefore, be possible to represent reactions by writing an equation which balances. The ability to write an equation for a reaction is the first step towards understanding that reaction.
Zinc will react with hydrochloric acid to form a solution of zinc chloride. During the course of the reaction hydrogen gas will be given off. (NB: Hydrochloric acid is a com-

bination of hydrogen chloride and water, but as the water is not changed in the reaction it need not be written in the equation.) With this information it is possible to write down the names of the substances involved in the reaction (the *reactants*) and the *products* of the reaction together with their chemical formulae: thus

Zinc + hydrogen chloride forms zinc chloride and hydrogen gas

$$Zn + HCl \rightarrow ZnCl_2 + H_2$$

The atoms present in the reactants and products of this reaction are:

zinc + hydrogen + chlorine → zinc + chlorine + hydrogen

$$1 + 1 + 1 \rightarrow 1 + 2 + 2$$

The products of this reaction contain twice as many atoms of hydrogen and chlorine as did the reactants. In other words, the equation does not balance so something is wrong somewhere. If the equation is to balance there need to be twice as many atoms of hydrogen and chloride (or twice as many molecules of hydrogen chloride) than there are atoms of zinc to start with. The equation will then read:

$$Zn + 2HCl \rightarrow ZnCl_2 + H_2$$

Although the formula of the reactants and products cannot be altered, the relative proportions can. In the above reaction atoms are neither gained nor lost (created nor destroyed) and the equation balances.

The physical states of the reactants and products (s:solid, l:liquid, g:gas, aq:aqueous solution) can be included in brackets after the formula if required:

$$Zn(s) + 2HCl(aq) \rightarrow ZnCl_2(aq) + H_2$$

A balanced equation will therefore provide information regarding:
- The formulae of reactants and products.
- The physical states of reactants and products.
- The quantities of reactants in proportion to products.

Balancing equations is not, therefore, merely an interesting academic exercise de-

signed to confuse and frustrate students! Scientists can use formulae and equations to calculate the quantities of the reactants and products of any given reaction. This information can be used to determine such things as the amount of raw material needed to produce a given quantity of a product (goods or power). They can also be used to forecast the nature and volume of any waste products that might evolve during the process. Industrial examples of the uses of such calculations include:
- Determining the amount of salt (NaCl) needed to produce 100 tonnes of chlorine (Cl)
- The volume of oxygen (O_2) needed to burn 100 g of methane (CH_4).
- The volume of carbon dioxide (CO_2) produced when 100 g of methane is burned.
- The volume of 10 per cent saline solution needed to recover all of the silver from 1 kg of an alloy containing 2 per cent silver.

Equilibrium Reactions

In many reactions when reactants combine to form products the process is complete and the reaction is said to be *irreversible*. For many reactions, however, there is a tendency for products to *decompose* (break down) and become reactants again. Such reactions are said to be *reversible*. In writing chemical equations such reactions are indicated by double arrows:

$$3H_2 + N_2 \rightleftharpoons 2NH_3$$

A state of equilibrium (or balance) is reached when the rate of reaction is equal in both ways, that is to say the original substances are reacting at the same rate as the newly formed substances. To maintain chemical equilibrium, the temperature and pressure must be kept constant and no substance must be added or removed, in other words the system must be kept *closed*.

If two substances A and B react to form two substances C + D a state of equilibrium is denoted by the balanced equation:

$$A + B \rightleftharpoons C + D$$

Any reaction has a theoretical maximum yield which is expressed as an *equilibrium constant*.

Requirements for a Reaction to Occur

For a reaction to occur the reactant molecules must meet and collide. This is clearly affected by the concentration of reactants. The more molecules present the more likely they are to meet and collide.

In any reaction there will be an overall energy change, so molecules must meet with enough energy to react. Increasing the temperature (and hence the amount of energy available) increases the chance of a reaction occurring. A catalyst will assist by reducing the energy requirements of the reactants.

The *equilibrium constant* or the *theoretical maximum yield* must be sufficiently large to allow the reaction to occur.

Naming Organic Compounds

Most well-known organic chemicals have two names. Nurses will be familiar with many of these, for example, acetone. Nurses may also wonder why some of these old common names are being replaced with new unfamiliar ones: acetone, for example, is now called propanone.

Systematic Nomenclature

Since 1948 efforts have been made to systemize the names of organic chemicals. The 'new' names are derived from an internationally agreed system of nomenclature. This system gives a completely descriptive name to every organic substance, one which permits only one structural formula to be written for it. Generally nurses will not need to write formulae, the brief explanation which follows is simply intended to help them understand the system.

Aliphatic Compounds

Every name consists of a *root*, a *suffix* and as many *prefixes* as necessary. The simplest group of hydrocarbons, for example, is the alkanes, which have a suffix 'ane'. The root is determined by the number of carbon atoms in the longest carbon chain. Having identified the longest chain it is then necessary to identify various functional groups and to name them. *Table* 2 shows the roots of aliphatic nomenclature. *Table* 3 shows some common functional groups.

Aromatic Compounds

The names of aromatic compounds are derived from benzene or similar aromatic hydrocarbons. The carbon atoms in the benzene ring are numbered from the carbon atom to which the principal group is attached. Some examples of systematic nomenclature for aliphatic and aromatic compounds follow.

Alkanes

Single bonds (saturated hydrocarbons), suffix 'ane'. To find the longest chain the carbon atoms are numbered from one end, ensuring that the lowest number possible is used to indicate the position of the side chain.

2,4,dimethyl hexane

$$^6CH_3 - {}^5CH_2 - {}^4CH - {}^3CH_2 - {}^2CH - {}^1CH_3$$
$$\qquad\qquad\quad | \qquad\qquad |$$
$$\qquad\qquad CH_3 \qquad\quad CH_3$$

3 ethyl, 5 methyl octane

$$^1CH_3 - {}^2CH_2 - {}^3CH - {}^4CH_2 - {}^5CH - CH_3$$
$$\qquad\qquad\quad | \qquad\qquad\qquad |$$
$$\qquad\qquad CH_2 - CH_3 \; {}^6CH_2 - {}^7CH_2 - {}^8CH_3$$

This can also be written as:

$$\qquad\qquad\qquad\qquad CH_3$$
$$\qquad\qquad\qquad\qquad |$$
$$^1CH_3 - {}^2CH_2 - {}^3CH - {}^4CH_2 - {}^5CH - {}^6CH_2 - {}^7CH_2 - {}^8CH_3$$
$$\qquad\qquad\quad |$$
$$\qquad\qquad CH_2 - CH_3$$

NB: Attached groups must be written in alphabetical order with their corresponding number.

3 ethyl, 2 methyl pentane

$$\qquad\qquad\qquad CH_3$$
$$\qquad\qquad\qquad |$$
$$CH_3 - {}^4CH_2 - {}^3CH - {}^2CH - {}^1CH_3$$
$$\qquad\qquad\quad |$$
$$\qquad\qquad CH_2 - CH_3$$

Alkenes

This group contains double-bonded carbon atoms and has the suffix 'ene'.

ethene

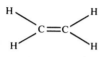

The multiple bonds in the chain are given the lowest number, they take precedence over the attached groups.

2 ethyl but-1-ene

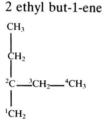

hex-3-ene

$^1CH_3$—$^2CH_2$—^3CH═^4CH—$^5CH_2$—$^6CH_3$

Alkynes

This group contains triple carbon bonds and have the suffix 'yne'.

ethyne (acetylene)

H—C≡C—H

but-1-yne

$^4CH_3$—$^3CH_2$—^2C≡^1CH

propyne

CH_3—C≡CH

aromatic systems (based on benzene C_6H_6)

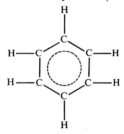

Hydroxyl Compounds

The suffix here is 'ol'.

Primary alcohols
methanol (methyl alcohol)

CH_3——OH

ethanol (ethyl alcohol)

CH_3——CH_2—OH

propan-1-ol

CH_3—CH_2—CH_2—OH

Secondary and tertiary alcohols

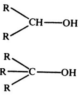

R = alkyl group e.g.

propan-2-ol

CH_3——CH—OH
           |
          CH_3

-2 methyl propan-2-ol

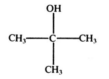

Halides

Compounds containing chlorine (suffix chloride), bromine (suffix bromide) etc.

Alkyl halides

chloroethane (ethyl chloride)

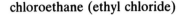

CH_3——CH_2——Cl

2 bromopropane

CH_3——CH——CH_3

Br

Aryl halide

bromobenzene

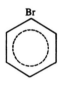

Br

Aldehydes

Suffix 'anal'.

methanal (formaldehyde)

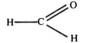

ethanal (acetaldehyde)

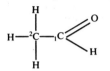

propanal

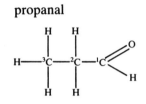

Amines

Suffix 'ylamine'.

Primary amines

methylamine

CH_3——NH_2

ethylamine

CH_3——CH_2——NH_2

Secondary amines

diethylamine

CH_3——CH_2

CH_3——CH_2 ⟩NH

Tertiary amines

triethylamine

CH_3——CH_2
CH_2——CH_2 ⟩N
CH_3——CH_2

Ketones

Suffix 'anone'.

ethanone

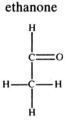

propanone

CH_3——C——CH_3

O

Carboxylic Acids
Those with longer chains are called fatty acids. Suffix 'anoic'.

methanoic acid (formic acid)

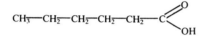

ethanoic acid (acetic acid)

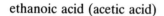

hexanoic acid

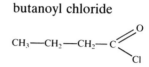

Esters
methyl ethanoic (methyl acetate)

Acid Chlorides
Suffix 'anoyl chloride'.

ethanoyl chloride

butanoyl chloride

Acid Amides
Suffix 'anamide'.

ethanamide

butanamide

Table 2 Alkanes and roots of aliphatic compounds

Alkane		Root	No. of carbon atoms in chain
Methane	CH_4	meth	1
Ethane	CH_3—CH_3	eth	2
Propane	CH_3—CH_2—CH_3	prop	3
Butane	CH_3—CH_2—CH_2—CH_3	but	4
Pentane	CH_3—CH_2—CH_2—CH_2—CH_3	pent	5
Hexane	CH_3—CH_2—CH_2—CH_2—CH_2—CH_3	hex	6
Heptane	CH_3—CH_2—CH_2—CH_2—CH_2—CH_2—CH_3	hep	7
Octane	CH_3—CH_2—CH_2—CH_2—CH_2—CH_2—CH_2—CH_3	oct	8

Table 3 Some common functional groups

Functional group	Structure	Prefix	Suffix
Single bond			ane
Double bond	$C{=}C$		ene
Triple bond	$C{\equiv}C$		yne
Halogen (X= Cl,Br, or I)		chloro bromo iodo	chloride bromide iodode
Amine		amino	amine
Hydroxyl		hydroxy	ol
Carbonyl		oxo	al (in aldehydes) one (in ketones)
Carboxyl		carboxy	oic acid
Acid chloride			oyl chloride
Amide		amido	amide
Ester			oate
Nitrile	$-C{\equiv}N$	cyano	nitrile

Glossary

abscissa   The measurement on a graph made along or parallel to the horizontal axis.

absorption   The taking up of a material by the skin, mucous membrane etc.

acid base balance   The correct ratio of hydrogen (H) ions and carboxyl (OH) ions in the blood.

activation energy   The minimum energy required by an atom in order for it to react.

adsorption   The adhesion of films of solids, liquids or gases to the surface of solid bodies.

alpha particle   A helium nucleus emitted by an atom during radioactive decay.

amino acid   The simple molecule from which proteins are synthesized or into which proteins can be broken down.

amplitude   The maximum displacement of a vibration or wave.

anabolism   The process of synthesis in the living cell.

anion   A negatively charged ion.

atom   The smallest unit of an element which can take part in a chemical reaction.

atomic number   The number of protons in a nucleus; in a neutral atom it is also equal to the number of orbiting electrons.

ATP   Adenosine triphisulphate, a substance involved in nucleic acid metabolism and energy production in the cell.

beta particle   A fast electron emitted by the nucleus of an atom during radioactive decay.

buffer   A compound with power to combine with either an acid or a base to help maintain acid base balance.

calorie   The unit of the quantity of heat.

carbohydrate   A group of chemical compounds composed of carbon, hydrogen and oxygen only and which include the sugars, starch and cellulose.

catabolism   The process of the breakdown of molecules in the cell.

catalyst   An agent which changes the rate of a chemical reaction without itself being used up or changed.

cathode   A negative electrode.

cation   A positively charged ion which is attracted towards the negatively charged cathode during electrolysis.

chemical symbol   The representation of an atom of a particular element.

co-enzyme   A relatively small organic substance which is essential to the action of some enzymes.

colloid   A substance which diffuses slowly or not at all.

compound   A substance formed by the chemical combination of two or more atoms of different elements in definite proportions by weight.

conjugated protein   A simple protein united with another compound such as a pigment or a carbohydrate.

crystalloid   A substance which, when in solution, can pass through a semi-permeable membrane. Opposite of colloid.

cycle   A complete set of movements in a vibration or wave.

cytoplasm   The protoplasm of a living cell which is outside the nucleus.

decay   The decrease of some factor with time.

Can be applied for instance to the amplitude of a vibration and to radioactivity.

decibel   The unit of sound measurement.

deuteron   The nucleus of a deuterium atom sometimes emitted during radioactive decay.

dialysis   The selective diffusion of a substance through a semi-permeable membrane for the separation of colloids from other dissolved substances.

diffusion   A spreading or mixing of molecules of a gas or a substance in solution so that the solution becomes uniform in concentration throughout.

DNA   Deoxyribonucleic acid. A high molecular weight substance found in the nucleus of cells, it is the hereditary material of most living organisms.

electric field   The region around an electrical charge in which a force will be exerted on any charged particle.

electrode   A charged substance which acts as a conductor allowing an electric current to enter or leave an electrolyte in electrolysis. An anode is a positive electrode and a cathode a negative one.

electrolysis   The decomposition of a substance by the passage of an electric current.

electrolyte   A substance which ionizes in solution.

electron   A sub-atomic particle which carries a negative electrical charge.

electronic configuration   The number and arrangement of orbiting electrons in an atom.

element   A pure substance which cannot be broken down into any other element and which contains only atoms of the same atomic number.

endothermic reaction   A reaction which uses heat energy.

energy   The power to do work or to produce change.

enzyme   A protein which acts as a catalyst in living organisms; almost all enzymes are highly specific so large numbers of them exist.

equation, chemical   A way of expressing the reactants and products of a chemical reaction.

ester   A product formed by the interaction of an acid and an alcohol.

exothermic reaction   A reaction in which heat is produced.

fatty acids   The basic units from which lipids are formed.

fission, nuclear   The splitting of a nucleus into two nuclei of comparable size.

force   A push or pull which acts on an object by causing it to move, slow down, speed up or stop.

formula   A representation of the ratio of the atoms of each element in a compound. *Molecular formulae* give the actual number of the atoms of each element present in the molecule.

frequency   The number of vibrations or waves that occurs in a second.

fusion, nuclear   The joining together of two or more nuclei to form one nucleus.

gamma rays   High frequency radiation emitted by a nuclide during radioactive decay.

glycine   A simple amino acid.

half-life   The time taken for half of a given sample of a radioactive nuclide to decay.

hydrocarbon   A compound composed only of carbon and hydrogen atoms.

hydrolysis   The splitting of a large molecule into two or more smaller ones with the addition of one molecule of water for each molecule formed.

hypothesis   An assertion put forward as a basis for research.

inert gas   The Noble gases, helium, neon, argon, krypton, xenon and radon, which are all chemically unreactive.

ion   An atom which has become electrically charged through the loss or gain of one or more electrons.

ionize   To dissociate a compound into ions.

irradiate   To affect by electromagnetic waves.

isomer   One of two or more chemical compounds with the same molecular formula but different arrangement of atoms and so possessing different properties.

isotopes   Atoms of the same element which carry the same number of protons but a different number of neutrons. They have the same atomic number but a different mass number.

isotonic Having the same tension or pressure.

ketone A compound formed by the oxidation of a secondary alcohol.

latent period The length of time which elapses between a stimulus and a response.

law, scientific An explanation for a given set of facts which is generally held to be correct within its limits.

lipids Fats and fat-like substances.

logarithm A number expressed as the power of another number.

magnetic field The space around a magnet in which a force can be detected.

manometer An instrument for measuring pressure.

mass number The total number of nucleons in a nucleus.

meniscus The curved surface of a liquid in a vessel.

metabolism Biological changes, the combination of anabolism and catabolism.

micro-organism Any microscopic life form such as bacteria.

molar solution A solution containing 1 mole of solute in 1 litre of a solution.

molecule The smallest portion of a substance capable of existing independently and still retaining the properties of the original substance.

natural frequency The frequency at which an object will vibrate if left free to do so.

natural vibration Once started, the vibration of an object with no outside interference.

neutrino A stable element particle with no electrical charge. It is known to exist in two forms; the neutrino, which, during radioactive decay, is emitted with positive positrons and the anti-neutrino, which is emitted with negative electrons.

neutron A sub-atomic particle with zero charge. Present in all atomic nuclei except normal hydrogen.

nucleic acid The giant molecules DNA and RNA which are found in all living things.

nucleon A proton or a neutron, constituents of the nucleus.

nucleotide A sub-unit of a nucleic acid.

nucleus, atomic The positively charged core of an atom which contains the neucleons (protons and neutrons).

nucleus, cell A highly differentiated body surrounded by a membrane which is found within the cytoplasm of most biological cells (plants and animals). It contains the chromosomes and is the organelle of reproduction.

ordinate The measurement on a graph made along or parallel to the vertical axis.

organ A structure composed of two or more tissues and one which has a specific function.

organelle A part of the living cell which is structurally and functionally discrete and often bounded by a membrane.

organism A single living thing, plant or animal.

osmosis Diffusion through a membrane from a lower to a more concentrated solution.

osmotic pressure The pressure generated by osmosis.

pepsin An enzyme present in the gastric juices.

Periodic Table of the Elements The arrangement of the elements in order of increasing atomic number and with the elements which have similar properties grouped together.

pH value The hydrogen ion concentration of a solution expressed as a negative logarithm.

plasma (phys.) Ionized gas molecules.

plasma (biol.) The liquid portion of blood.

plasma membrane The outer membrane of a cell which possesses selective permeability.

positron A positive electron of the same mass and energy as a negative electron; the electrical charge is of the same magnitude.

precipitate An insoluble substance formed in a solution as a result of chemical change.

proton A sub-atomic particle with a positive charge.

protoplasm The matter of which all biological cells consist.

purines and pyrimidines The basic units of nucleotides.

radiation Emission of waves such as light, radio, sound, from a vibrating source.

reciprocal   The inverse of any number. For example, the reciprocal of 2 is 1/2 of 6 is 1/6.

scalar   A quantity of size only.

somatic   Pertaining to the body.

substrate   A substance on which an enzyme acts.

surface tension   The net force exerted at the surface of a liquid due to the unequal intermolecular forces acting on surface molecules.

synthesis   The formation of a compound from elements or simpler compounds.

theory   An assertion which explains certain facts but which is not claimed to be totally correct.

tissue   An aggregate of similar cells.

tissue fluid   Fluid found in tissue spaces, lymph.

transmutation   Change of one element into another by a process of radioactive decay.

valency   The combining power of an atom or group of atoms.

vector   A quantity which has both magnitude (size) and direction.

wavelength   The distance between two consecutive positions in a wave in which movements are exactly the same shape.

zwitterion   A dipolar compound such as an amino acid which contains a positive amino group and a negative carboxyl group.

The Greek Alphabet

A	α	Alpha	I	ι	Iota	P	ρ	Rho
B	β	Beta	K	κ	Kappa	Σ	σ	Sigma
Γ	γ	Gamma	Λ	λ	Lambda	T	τ	Tau
Δ	δ	Delta	M	μ	Mu	Y	υ	Upsilon
E	ε	Epsilon	N	ν	Nu	Φ	ϕ	Phi
Z	ζ	Zeta	Ξ	ξ	Xi	X	χ	Chi
H	η	Eta	O	o	Omicron	Ψ	ψ	Psi
Θ	θ	Theta	Π	π	Pi	Ω	ω	Omega

Index